Clinician's Guide to Laboratory Medicine

P•O•C•K•E•T

LEXI-COMP

Clinician's Guide to Laboratory Medicine

P•O•C•K•E•T

Samir P. Desai, MD

Assistant Professor of Medicine
Baylor College of Medicine
Houston, TX

Staff Physician
Michael E. DeBakey VA Medical Center
Houston, TX

LEXI-COMP INC
Hudson, Ohio

DEDICATION

To Teja

NOTICE

This handbook is intended to serve as a useful reference and not as a complete laboratory testing resource. The explosion of information in many directions, in multiple scientific disciplines, with advances in laboratory techniques, and continuing evolution of knowledge requires constant scholarship. The authors, editors, reviewers, contributors, and publishers cannot be responsible for the continued currency of the information or for any errors or omissions in this book or for any consequences arising therefrom. Because of the dynamic nature of laboratory medicine as a discipline, readers are advised that decisions regarding diagnosis and treatment must be based on the independent judgment of the clinician. The editors are not responsible for any inaccuracy of quotation or for any false or misleading implication that may arise due to the text.

LEXI-COMP

1100 Terex Road
Hudson, Ohio 44236
(330) 650-6506

ISBN 1-59195-072-4

CLINICIAN'S GUIDE TO LABORATORY MEDICINE - POCKET

TABLE OF CONTENTS

ALGORITHMS

ABOUT THE AUTHOR

Samir P. Desai, MD

Dr. Samir Desai serves on the faculty of the Baylor College of Medicine in the Department of Medicine. Dr. Desai has educated and mentored both medical students and residents, work for which he has received teaching awards.

Dr. Desai is the author of the popular *101 Biggest Mistakes 3rd Year Medical Students Make And How to Avoid Them*, a book that has helped students reach their full potential during the third year of medical school. In the book, *The Residency Match: 101 Biggest Mistakes And How To Avoid Them*, Dr. Desai shows applicants how to avoid commonly made mistakes during the residency application process. In the *Internal Medicine Clerkship: 150 Biggest Mistakes And How To Avoid Them*, students can not only learn about the errors their predecessors made but also avoid these pitfalls, which is crucial for success during this very important rotation.

Dr. Desai conceived and authored the "Clinician's Guide Series," a series of books dedicated to providing clinicians with practical approaches to commonly encountered problems. The *Clinician's Guide to Laboratory Medicine* and *Clinician's Guide to Diagnosis* have become popular books for healthcare professionals, providing a step-by-step approach to laboratory test interpretation and symptom evaluation, respectively. The *Clinician's Guide to Internal Medicine* offers quick access to key information that is needed in the care of patients with a wide variety of medical problems.

Dr. Desai is also the founder of www.md2b.net, a website committed to helping today's medical student become tomorrow's doctor. Founded in 2002, www.md2b.net is dedicated to providing medical students with the tools needed to tackle the challenges of the clinical years of medical school.

After completing his residency training in Internal Medicine at Northwestern University in Chicago, Illinois, Dr. Desai had the opportunity of serving as chief medical resident. He received his MD degree from the Wayne State University School of Medicine in Detroit, Michigan, graduating first in his class.

PREFACE

The interpretation of laboratory tests is difficult for many clinicians. This is especially true for clinicians-in-training who often feel ill at ease when they are faced with abnormal lab tests. Much of this anxiety has to do with the fact the currently available laboratory medicine textbooks, many of which are excellent resources, are either comprehensive tomes from which it is difficult to access information rapidly or handbooks which fail to provide guidance.

Unlike the comprehensive tomes of laboratory medicine, the *Clinician's Guide to Laboratory Medicine: Pocket* is portable and can easily be carried in any coat pocket. This is ideal for use at times when access to a larger laboratory medicine textbook is not available. Unlike most of the handbooks of laboratory medicine, the *Clinician's Guide to Laboratory Medicine: Pocket* does much more than just list a differential diagnosis for an abnormal lab test; it provides the essential information that clinicians need to approach commonly encountered laboratory test abnormalities.

Although the information present in this book has been extracted from the third edition of the *Clinician's Guide to Laboratory Medicine: A Practical Approach*, it can certainly be used independently of this larger handbook. There may be times, however, when the clinician requires more information in which case the clinician may wish to turn to this larger handbook or to another more definitive resource.

In summary, the *Clinician's Guide to Laboratory Medicine: Pocket* is not intended to take the place of the more specialized textbooks of laboratory medicine but to complement these resources by providing practical information in a concise, portable handbook that is easy to use at the point of care. I hope that the *Clinician's Guide to Laboratory Medicine: Pocket* becomes your companion both in the hospital and office setting, providing you, the clinician, with the tools necessary to tackle even the most challenging laboratory test results that await you.

— Samir Desai, MD

ACKNOWLEDGMENTS

The *Clinician's Guide to Laboratory Medicine: Pocket* is the most recent addition to Lexi-Comp's "Clinician's Guide Series" which also includes the *Clinician's Guide to Laboratory Medicine: A Practical Approach,* the *Clinician's Guide to Diagnosis: A Practical Approach*, and the *Clinician's Guide to Internal Medicine: A Practical Approach.* As the books' writer, I have had the great opportunity to work with a number of individuals at Lexi-Comp, Inc, all of whom have played key roles in the development of the *Clinician's Guide to Laboratory Medicine: Pocket.* This has truly been a team effort and I thank the entire staff at Lexi-Comp for letting me be a part of their first-class team.

I would like to express my appreciation to Robert D. Kerscher, president of Lexi-Comp, for his continued support of not only this book but also the entire "Clinician's Guide Series." I remain indebted to Lynn Coppinger for the time, effort, and energy she has expended in the development of this book. Matt Kerscher, product manager, deserves special thanks as well. It is through his tireless efforts that the 'Clinician's Guide Series' continues to grow. I would also like to thank Tracey Reinecke for her assistance with the cover design, Jeanne Wilson for her work on the web page product, and Dave Marcus for his expertise in indexing.

Finally, I would like to thank Dr. Jeff Bates for his insight during the preparation of this book. I am lucky to have him not only as a colleague but also a good friend. I appreciate all of his help with this book as well as the other titles in the "Clinician's Guide Series."

— Samir Desai, MD

HEMATOLOGY

COMPLETE BLOOD COUNT

The complete blood count (CBC) is not a single test but a battery of tests which includes the following:

- White blood cell count
- White blood cell count differential
- Hemoglobin
- Hematocrit
- Red blood cell count
- Red blood cell indices
- Platelet count

The CBC is the standard test for the evaluation of red blood cells, white blood cells, and platelets. Most laboratories use automated counters to determine the various components of the CBC.

HEMOGLOBIN / HEMATOCRIT

Hemoglobin refers to the concentration of hemoglobin in whole blood. Hematocrit is defined as the percentage of whole blood that is comprised of red blood cells. Hemoglobin and hematocrit essentially provide similar information. Either value, if low, confirms the presence of anemia. A useful relationship between hemoglobin and hematocrit is as follows:

$$\text{Hemoglobin} \times 3 = \text{Hematocrit}$$

Because this is a consistent relationship, it is not necessary to report the results of both hemoglobin and hematocrit. It is a matter of preference as to which one is used.

Causes of falsely elevated hemoglobin levels include lipemic plasma and marked increases in the white blood cell count (>50,000/mm^3). Causes of falsely high hematocrit levels include cryoproteins, giant platelets, and marked increases in the white blood cell count.

RED BLOOD CELL INDICES

Red blood cell indices include mean corpuscular volume (MCV), mean corpuscular hemoglobin (MCH), and mean corpuscular hemoglobin concentration (MCHC).

Mean Corpuscular Volume (MCV)

MCV is a measure of the volume or size of the average red blood cell. The MCV is often used in the evaluation of anemia. Based upon the patient's MCV, the anemia may be classified as microcytic, normocytic, or macrocytic, as follows:

- *Microcytosis*: A decrease in the red blood cell volume (<80 fL)
- *Normocytosis*: Normal red blood cell volume (80-96 fL)
- *Macrocytosis*: An elevation in red blood cell volume (>96 fL)

The MCV is typically determined by the use of an automated cell counter. These cell counters may yield erroneous values in the following conditions:

- Agglutination of red blood cells in the presence of cold agglutinins or cryoglobulins
- Significantly increased white blood cell count
- Plasma hyperosmolality

Remember that the MCV is a measure of average cell size. Individual red blood cells may vary in size but the MCV may not reflect this. For example, a patient can have two etiologies contributing to anemia. If one etiology is characterized by microcytosis and the other by macrocytosis, the MCV may fall in the normocytic range, as automated counters estimate average cell size. A review of the peripheral blood smear, however, will reveal a mixed population of cells, emphasizing the importance of looking at every peripheral blood smear!

When the MCV is high in the absence of anemia, the clinician should consider alcoholism, megaloblastic anemia, and drug-induced etiologies. A low MCV in the absence of anemia should prompt concern for thalassemia minor or polycythemia vera.

Mean Corpuscular Hemoglobin (MCH)

The MCH refers to the weight of hemoglobin in the average red blood cell. The reference range for MCH is 26-34 pg.

Mean Corpuscular Hemoglobin Concentration (MCHC)

The MCHC is a measure of the amount of hemoglobin present in the average red blood cell when compared to its size. In men, the reference range for MCHC is 31-37 g/dL. In women, the reference range is 30-36 g/dL. Fifty percent of patients with hereditary spherocytosis have an MCHC >36 g/dL.

RED BLOOD CELL DISTRIBUTION WIDTH

Normally, most red blood cells are equal in size. In many types of anemia, however, there is variability in red blood cell size, also known as anisocytosis. The red blood cell distribution width, or RDW, is a measure of this variability. This difference in size between cells is reflected in the RDW. Any process that leads to a wide variation in cell size will manifest with an increased RDW.

Causes of Microcytic Anemia Associated With Normal RDW

- Thalassemia minor
- Anemia of chronic disease
- Some hemoglobinopathy traits

Causes of Microcytic Anemia Associated With High RDW

- Iron deficiency
- Hemoglobin H disease
- Some anemia of chronic disease
- Some thalassemia minor
- Fragmentation hemolysis

Causes of Normocytic Anemia Associated With Normal RDW

- Anemia of chronic disease
- Hereditary spherocytosis
- Some hemoglobinopathy traits
- Acute bleeding

Causes of Normocytic Anemia Associated With High RDW

- Early or partially treated iron or vitamin deficiency
- Sickle cell anemia

Causes of Macrocytic Anemia Associated With Normal RDW

- Aplastic anemia
- Some myelodysplasias

Causes of Macrocytic Anemia Associated With High RDW

- Vitamin B_{12} deficiency
- Folate deficiency
- Autoimmune hemolytic anemia
- Cold agglutinin disease
- Some myelodysplasias
- Liver disease
- Thyroid disease
- Alcohol

PERIPHERAL BLOOD SMEAR

Inspection of the peripheral blood smear will provide the clinician with the opportunity to describe abnormalities in the size, shape, and number of red blood cells, white blood cells, and platelets. Variation in cell size is known as anisocytosis whereas variation in cell shape is referred to as poikilocytosis. It is not sufficient to merely take note of anisocytosis or poikilocytosis on the peripheral blood smear; rather, the clinician should strive to describe the abnormalities present.

Abnormalities of Red Blood Cell Shape

Spherocyte: Autoimmune hemolysis, hereditary spherocytosis, hemoglobinopathies, artifact

Tear drop cells (dacrocyte): Myeloid metaplasia with myelofibrosis, myelophthisic process, thalassemia, pernicious anemia

Target cell (codocyte): Chronic liver disease, thalassemia, hemoglobin C, S, or D disease, iron deficiency, splenectomy

Macroovalocyte: Megaloblastic anemia

Stomatocyte: Hereditary stomatocytosis, alcoholic cirrhosis

Schistocyte: Microangiopathic hemolytic anemia, heart valve hemolysis, severe burns

Echinocyte (burr cell): Kidney disease, heart disease, untreated hypothyroidism, artifact, bleeding ulcers, gastric carcinoma

Acanthocyte (spur cell): Liver disease, abetalipoproteinemia, hypothyroidism, vitamin E deficiency, splenectomy

Sickle cell (drepanocyte): Sickle cell anemia, other hemoglobinopathies

Rouleaux formation: Multiple myeloma, chronic liver disease, hypergammaglobulinemia, artifact

Agglutinated red blood cells: Cold agglutinin disease, artifact

Erythrocytic Inclusions

Howell-Jolly body: Splenectomy, hemolytic anemia, megaloblastic anemia

Basophilic stippling: Lead poisoning, thalassemia, splenectomy, hemolytic anemias

Cabot's ring: Megaloblastic anemia, thalassemia, splenectomy, hemolytic anemias

Pappenheimer body: Sickle cell anemia, thalassemia, megaloblastic anemia, sideroblastic anemia

Heinz body: Splenectomy, hemoglobinopathies, hemolytic anemia (G6PD deficiency)

WBC Abnormalities

Hypersegmented PMNs: Megaloblastic anemia

Hypogranular neutrophils: Chronic myelogenous leukemia (some cases)

Auer rods: Acute myelogenous leukemia

Pseudo-Pelger-Huët anomaly: Myelodysplastic syndrome

Intraleukocytic microorganisms: Ehrlichia species

Left shift (increase in band %): Consider bacterial infection

Toxic granulations / toxic vacuolation / Döhle bodies: Acute infection (typically bacterial)

RETICULOCYTE COUNT

Determination of the reticulocyte count is an essential part of the evaluation of the anemic patient. Reticulocytes are young red blood cells that contain residual RNA.

The reticulocyte count reflects the ability of the bone marrow to produce mature red blood cells. In the absence of anemia, a normal reticulocyte count varies from 1% to 2%. In an anemic patient, an increase in the reticulocyte count provides evidence that the bone marrow is adequately responding to the anemia.

When anemia develops, the bone marrow should respond with an increase in the reticulocyte count in an effort to maintain the hemoglobin level. The absence of an increase in the reticulocyte count reflects an inability of the bone marrow to compensate for the anemia. The laboratory will report the reticulocyte count as a percentage of the total red blood cell count. To interpret the reticulocyte count, several corrections must be made. The first correction involves adjusting the reticulocyte count for the degree of anemia as shown below:

Reticulocyte % corrected = reticulocyte % reported x (patient's hematocrit) / 45

This calculation will yield the corrected reticulocyte count. To calculate the reticulocyte production index (RPI) from the corrected reticulocyte count, another correction must be made, as shown below:

RPI = reticulocyte % corrected / correction factor

The correction factor used in the RPI calculation varies depending upon the patient's hematocrit, as shown below:

Patient's hematocrit 40 to 45: Use 1.0 as correction factor

Patient's hematocrit 35 to 39: Use 1.5 as correction factor

Patient's hematocrit 25 to 34: Use 2.0 as correction factor

Patient's hematocrit 15 to 24: Use 2.5 as correction factor

Patient's hematocrit <15: Use 3.0 as correction factor

An RPI value <2 is indicative of inadequate bone marrow response while a level >2 suggests that the bone marrow is responding appropriately for the degree of anemia. There are many causes of RPI <2 but the only three causes of RPI >2 are acute blood loss, hemolysis, and response to therapy (eg, iron replacement in patient with iron deficiency anemia).

ANEMIA

Anemia is defined as a hemoglobin or hematocrit below the lower limit of normal. Anemia should always be considered a symptom or sign of an underlying disease. As such, it is never appropriate to ignore this important finding. When the presence of anemia is discovered, it is incumbent upon the clinician to determine the etiology. The approach to the patient with anemia is described in the algorithm on the next page.

ANEMIA

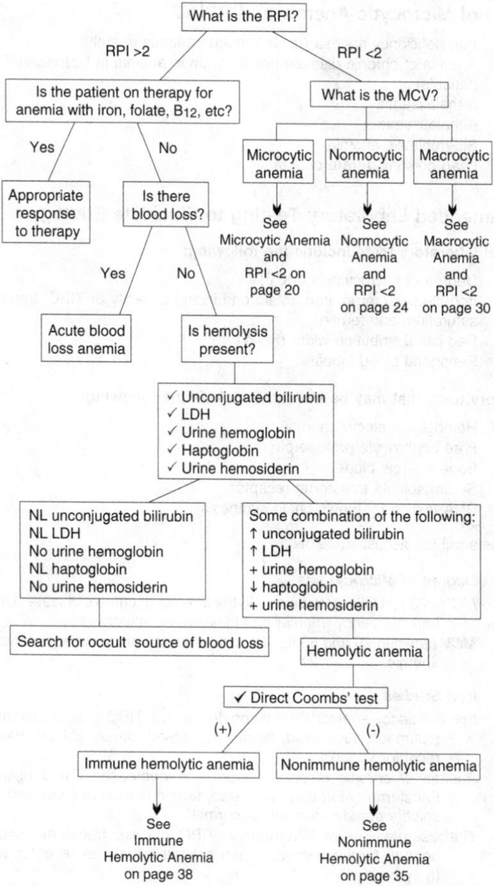
What is the RPI?
RPI >2
RPI <2
Is the patient on therapy for anemia with iron, folate, B12, etc?
Yes
No
Appropriate response to therapy
Is there blood loss?
Yes
No
Acute blood loss anemia
Is hemolysis present?
✓ Unconjugated bilirubin
✓ LDH
✓ Urine hemoglobin
✓ Haptoglobin
✓ Urine hemosiderin
NL unconjugated bilirubin
NL LDH
No urine hemoglobin
NL haptoglobin
No urine hemosiderin
Search for occult source of blood loss
Some combination of the following:
↑ unconjugated bilirubin
↑ LDH
+ urine hemoglobin
↓ haptoglobin
+ urine hemosiderin
Hemolytic anemia
✓ Direct Coombs' test
(+)
(-)
Immune hemolytic anemia
Nonimmune hemolytic anemia
See Immune Hemolytic Anemia on page 38
See Nonimmune Hemolytic Anemia on page 35
What is the MCV?
Microcytic anemia
Normocytic anemia
Macrocytic anemia
See Microcytic Anemia and RPI <2 on page 20
See Normocytic Anemia and RPI <2 on page 24
See Macrocytic Anemia and RPI <2 on page 30

MICROCYTIC ANEMIA AND RPI <2

Causes of Microcytic Anemia and RPI <2

- Iron deficiency anemia (most common anemia overall)
- Anemia of chronic disease (most common anemia in hospitalized patients)
- α-thalassemia
- β-thalassemia
- Sideroblastic anemia
- Lead poisoning (rare cause)

Recommended Laboratory Testing to Elucidate Etiology

Essential laboratory tests include the following:

- Degree of microcytosis (MCV)
- Iron studies (serum iron, total iron binding capacity or TIBC, transferrin saturation, and ferritin)
- Red cell distribution width (RDW)
- Peripheral blood smear

Laboratory tests that may be indicated include the following:

- Hemoglobin electrophoresis
- Free erythrocyte protoporphyrin
- Bone marrow biopsy
- Serum soluble transferrin receptor
- DNA testing for globin chain synthesis

These tests will be discussed below.

- ***Degree of Microcytosis***

  MCV <70 fL: Unlikely to be due to the anemia of chronic disease. Consider iron deficiency anemia and thalassemia minor.

  MCV between 70 and 80 fL: May be due to any of the causes of microcytic anemia.

- ***Iron Studies***

  Iron deficiency anemia: Serum iron decreased, TIBC increased, transferrin saturation decreased, ferritin decreased, serum soluble transferrin receptor variable

  Anemia of chronic disease: Serum iron decreased, TIBC decreased, transferrin saturation decreased, ferritin normal or increased, serum soluble transferrin receptor normal

  Thalassemia: Serum iron normal, TIBC normal, transferrin saturation normal, ferritin normal, serum soluble transferrin receptor variable (may be high)

Sideroblastic anemia: Serum iron increased, TIBC normal, transferrin saturation increased, ferritin increased, serum soluble transferrin receptor variable (may be high)

- ***Red Cell Distribution Width***

Causes of microcytic anemia associated with normal RDW: Thalassemia minor, anemia of chronic disease

Causes of microcytic anemia associated with high RDW: Iron deficiency anemia, anemia of chronic disease (some cases), thalassemia minor (some cases)

- ***Peripheral Blood Smear***

Iron deficiency anemia: Anisocytosis, poikilocytosis, microcytosis, hypochromia, target cells, pencil cells, variable platelet count

Anemia of chronic disease: Microcytosis, hypochromia

Thalassemia minor: Microcytosis, hypochromia, target cells, basophilic stippling

Sideroblastic anemia: Anisocytosis, poikilocytosis, microcytosis, hypochromia, basophilic stippling, dimorphic population, ± dysplastic WBC features

- ***Bone Marrow Biopsy***

Not needed in most cases of microcytic anemia

Perform if etiology remains unclear despite performance of the above tests

Absence of iron stores by Prussian blue staining = iron deficiency anemia

Increased numbers of ringed sideroblasts = sideroblastic anemia

- ***Hemoglobin Electrophoresis***

Hemoglobin electrophoresis is helpful in establishing a diagnosis of thalassemia minor. An elevated hemoglobin A2 supports the diagnosis of β-thalassemia minor. α-thalassemia minor cannot be diagnosed by hemoglobin electrophoresis. Although DNA testing is required for the definitive diagnosis of α-thalassemia minor, in usual clinical practice, the diagnosis is one of exclusion.

MICROCYTIC ANEMIA IN THE PATIENT WITH RPI <2

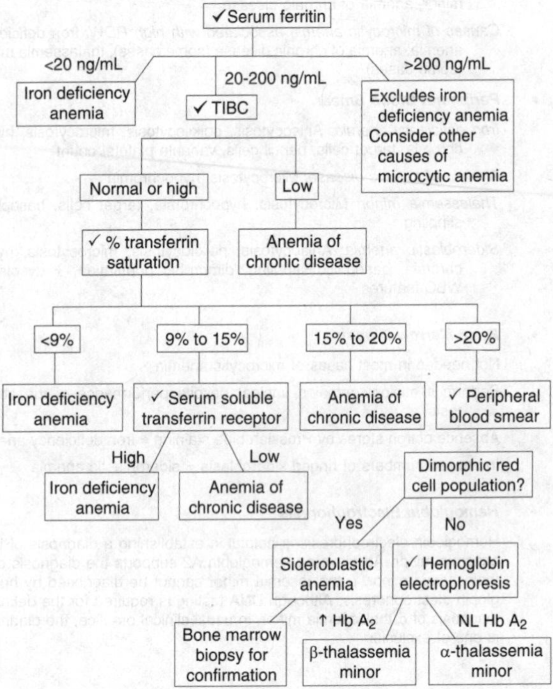
✓Serum ferritin
<20 ng/mL
Iron deficiency anemia
20-200 ng/mL
✓ TIBC
>200 ng/mL
Excludes iron deficiency anemia Consider other causes of microcytic anemia
Normal or high
Low
✓ % transferrin saturation
Anemia of chronic disease
<9%
9% to 15%
15% to 20%
>20%
Iron deficiency anemia
✓ Serum soluble transferrin receptor
Anemia of chronic disease
✓ Peripheral blood smear
High
Low
Iron deficiency anemia
Anemia of chronic disease
Dimorphic red cell population?
Yes
No
Sideroblastic anemia
✓ Hemoglobin electrophoresis
↑ Hb A2
NL Hb A2
Bone marrow biopsy for confirmation
β-thalassemia minor
α-thalassemia minor

NORMOCYTIC ANEMIA AND RPI <2

Causes of Normocytic Anemia and RPI <2

- Early iron deficiency anemia (most common anemia overall)
- Anemia of chronic disease (most common anemia in hospitalized patients)
- Anemia secondary to acute blood loss
- Aplastic anemia
- Pure red blood cell aplasia
- Myelodysplastic syndrome
- Myelophthisis
- Anemia of renal insufficiency
- Anemia of liver disease
- Anemia of endocrine disease
- Anemia associated with AIDS
- Sideroblastic anemia
- Megaloblastic anemia
- Mixed anemia

Recommended Laboratory Testing to Elucidate the Etiology

Essential laboratory tests include the following:

- Iron studies (serum iron, total iron binding capacity or TIBC, transferrin saturation, and serum ferritin)
- Peripheral blood smear
- Red blood cell distribution width
- Serum folate level
- Serum vitamin B_{12} level
- Serum BUN and creatinine
- Liver function tests

Laboratory tests that may be indicated include the following:

- Serum calcium (if hyperparathyroidism suspected)
- Thyroid function tests (if hyperthyroidism or hypothyroidism suspected)
- Cosyntropin stimulation test (if adrenal insufficiency suspected)
- HIV test (if anemia associated with AIDS suspected)
- Bone marrow biopsy

These tests will be discussed below.

- ***Peripheral Blood Smear***

  Decrease in white blood cells and / or platelets: Aplastic anemia, myelophthisis, myelodysplastic syndrome, megaloblastic anemia, anemia of liver disease

  Leukoerythroblastosis: Myelophthisis

  Abnormal white blood cells: Leukemia, lymphoma, myelodysplastic syndrome

  Rouleaux formation: Multiple myeloma

  Hypersegmented PMNs: Megaloblastic anemia

  Target cell: Anemia of liver disease

  Dimorphic population: Sideroblastic anemia

  Burr cell: Uremia (anemia of renal insufficiency)

- ***Red Blood Cell Distribution Width (RDW)***

  Causes of normocytic anemia associated with normal RDW: Anemia of chronic disease, anemia of acute blood loss, myelodysplastic syndrome

  Causes of normocytic anemia associated with elevated RDW: Early iron deficiency anemia, partially treated iron deficiency anemia, megaloblastic anemia, myelodysplastic syndrome, anemia of liver disease

- ***Iron Studies***

  Iron deficiency anemia: Serum iron decreased, TIBC increased, transferrin saturation decreased, ferritin decreased, serum soluble transferrin receptor variable

  Anemia of chronic disease: Serum iron decreased, TIBC decreased, transferrin saturation decreased, ferritin normal or increased, serum soluble transferrin receptor normal

- ***Serum Folate / Vitamin B_{12} Levels***
  Early megaloblastic anemia may present with normocytic anemia. Please see more information regarding the interpretation of serum folate and vitamin B_{12} levels *on page 28.*

- ***Serum BUN / Creatinine***

  Anemia of chronic renal insufficiency is a common cause of normocytic anemia. In general, the severity of the anemia correlates with the severity of the renal insufficiency. Major causes of anemia in these patients include decreased erythropoietin production, iron deficiency, folate deficiency, gastrointestinal blood loss, and decreased red blood cell survival.

- ***Liver Function Tests***

  Anemia of liver disease may be normocytic. Factors contributing the anemia of liver disease include anemia of chronic disease, folic acid deficiency, iron deficiency anemia, decreased red blood cell survival, toxic effects of alcohol, hemodilution, and hypersplenism.

- ***HIV Test***

  Causes of anemia in HIV / AIDS patients include anemia of chronic disease, suppression of bone marrow by HIV, medication-induced suppression of bone marrow, myelophthisis secondary to infection or malignancy, immune-mediated parvovirus infection causing pure red cell aplasia, and nutritional deficiency.

- ***Bone Marrow Biopsy***

  Required to establish the diagnosis of aplastic anemia, pure red cell aplasia, myelophthisis, and myelodysplastic syndrome. In general, bone marrow biopsy should be performed in every patient with normocytic anemia and RPI <2 in whom the etiology of the anemia remains unexplained despite the performance of the above tests.

NORMOCYTIC ANEMIA IN THE PATIENT WITH RPI <2

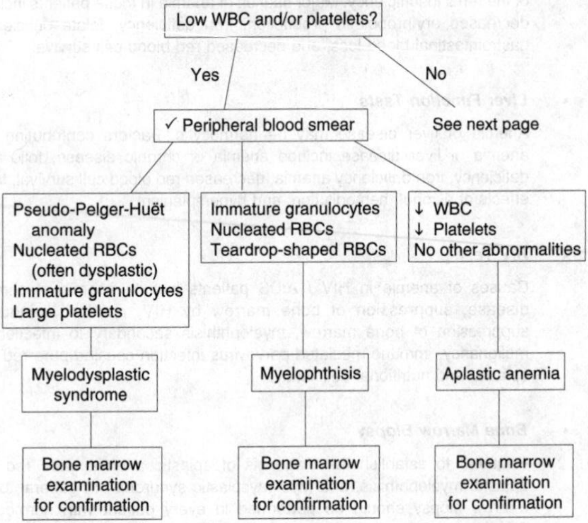
Low WBC and/or platelets?
Yes
No
✓ Peripheral blood smear
See next page
Pseudo-Pelger-Huët anomaly
Nucleated RBCs (often dysplastic)
Immature granulocytes
Large platelets
Immature granulocytes
Nucleated RBCs
Teardrop-shaped RBCs
↓ WBC
↓ Platelets
No other abnormalities
Myelodysplastic syndrome
Myelophthisis
Aplastic anemia
Bone marrow examination for confirmation
Bone marrow examination for confirmation
Bone marrow examination for confirmation

NORMOCYTIC ANEMIA IN THE PATIENT WITH RPI <2 *(continued)*

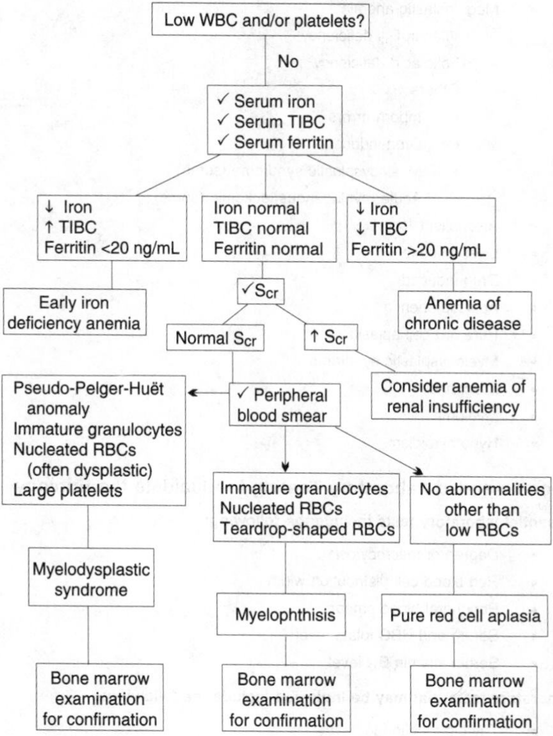
Low WBC and/or platelets?
No
✓ Serum iron
✓ Serum TIBC
✓ Serum ferritin
↓ Iron
↑ TIBC
Ferritin <20 ng/mL
Iron normal
TIBC normal
Ferritin normal
↓ Iron
↓ TIBC
Ferritin >20 ng/mL
Early iron deficiency anemia
✓Scr
Anemia of chronic disease
Normal Scr
↑ Scr
Pseudo-Pelger-Huët anomaly
Immature granulocytes
Nucleated RBCs (often dysplastic)
Large platelets
✓ Peripheral blood smear
Consider anemia of renal insufficiency
Immature granulocytes
Nucleated RBCs
Teardrop-shaped RBCs
No abnormalities other than low RBCs
Myelodysplastic syndrome
Myelophthisis
Pure red cell aplasia
Bone marrow examination for confirmation
Bone marrow examination for confirmation
Bone marrow examination for confirmation

S_{cr} = serum creatinine

MACROCYTIC ANEMIA AND RPI <2

Causes of Macrocytic Anemia and RPI <2

- Megaloblastic anemia
  - Vitamin B_{12} deficiency
  - Folic acid deficiency
  - Others
    - Inborn errors
    - Drug-induced
    - Myelodysplastic syndrome (some)
    - Acute myelogenous leukemia (some)
- Alcoholism
- Liver disease
- Drug-induced
- Aplastic anemia
- Pure red cell aplasia
- Myelodysplastic syndrome
- Pregnancy
- Myeloma
- Hypothyroidism

Recommended Laboratory Testing to Elucidate the Etiology

Essential laboratory tests include the following:

- Degree of macrocytosis
- Red blood cell distribution width
- Peripheral blood smear
- Serum and RBC folate level
- Serum vitamin B_{12} level

Laboratory tests that may be indicated include the following:

- Thyroid function tests
- Liver function tests
- Homocysteine level
- Methylmalonic acid level
- Schilling's test

- Anti-intrinsic factor antibodies
- Antiparietal cell antibodies
- Bone marrow biopsy

These tests will be discussed below.

- ***Degree of Macrocytosis***
  MCV >115 fL: Likely to be due to megaloblastic anemia
  MCV <115 fL: May be due to any of the causes of macrocytic anemia

- ***Red Blood Cell Distribution Width (RDW)***
  Causes of macrocytic anemia and RPI <2 associated with normal RDW: Aplastic anemia, some myelodysplasias
  Causes of macrocytic anemia and RPI <2 associated with high RDW: Vitamin B_{12} deficiency, folate deficiency, some myelodysplasias, liver disease, thyroid disease, alcohol

- ***Peripheral Blood Smear***
  Inspection of the peripheral blood smear is required in every patient with macrocytic anemia. The smear will help differentiate megaloblastic anemia from nonmegaloblastic anemia (see above). Hallmark finding of megaloblastic anemia is the hypersegmented PMN. Hypersegmented PMNs are said to be present if any of the following criteria are met:

  - At least one PMN containing ≥6 lobes
  - 5-lobe PMNs account for ≥5% of the total neutrophil count
  - Neutrophil lobe average ≥3.4

  Other peripheral blood smear findings of megaloblastic anemia include the following:

  - ± leukopenia
  - ± thrombocytopenia
  - Macroovalocytes
  - Anisopoikilocytosis
  - Nucleated red blood cells
  - Target cells
  - Schistocytes
  - Spherocytes
  - Erythrocytic inclusions (Howell-Jolly bodies, Cabot's rings, basophilic stippling)

  If hypersegmented PMNs (with or without other abnormalities of megaloblastic anemia) are present, serum folate and vitamin B_{12} levels are indicated. Although the absence of hypersegmented PMNs suggests a nonmegaloblastic cause of macrocytic anemia, most clinicians will still obtain serum folate and vitamin B_{12} levels. This is because, in some patients with megaloblastic anemia, the characteristic peripheral blood smear findings are lacking. In addition, many clinicians do not feel comfortable with their ability to recognize these findings.

- ***Serum Folate / Vitamin B_{12} Levels***

  When interpreting serum folate and vitamin B_{12} levels, the clinician should realize that low normal test results do not exclude the diagnosis of folate or B_{12} deficiency. Studies have shown that 10% of patients with clinically confirmed vitamin B_{12} deficiency have vitamin B_{12} levels in the low normal range (200-300 pg/mL). Twenty-five percent of patients with clinically confirmed folate deficiency have levels in the low normal range (2.5-5 ng/mL). When levels are in the low normal range, it is helpful to obtain homocysteine and methylmalonic acid levels.

  Vitamin B_{12} >300 pg/mL and folate >4 ng/mL: Vitamin B_{12} or folate deficiency unlikely (no need for homocysteine and methylmalonic acid levels)

  Vitamin B_{12} >300 pg/mL and folate <2 ng/mL: Folate deficiency (no need for homocysteine and methylmalonic acid levels)

  Vitamin B_{12} <200 pg/mL and folate >4 ng/mL: Vitamin B_{12} deficiency (no need for homocysteine and methylmalonic acid levels)

  Vitamin B_{12} 200-300 pg/mL and folate >4 ng/mL: Possible vitamin B_{12} deficiency (homocysteine and methylmalonic acid levels indicated)

  Vitamin B_{12} <200 pg/mL and folate <2 ng/mL: Isolated folate deficiency vs combined deficiency (homocysteine and methylmalonic acid levels indicated)

  Vitamin B_{12} >300 pg/mL and folate 2-4 ng/mL: Isolated folate deficiency vs another cause of anemia (homocysteine and methylmalonic acid levels indicated)

- ***Homocysteine / Methylmalonic Acid Levels***

  Normal methylmalonic acid level and increased homocysteine level: Folate deficiency likely (<5% have vitamin B_{12} deficiency)

  Increased methylmalonic acid level and increased homocysteine level: Vitamin B_{12} deficiency (cannot exclude folate deficiency)

  Normal methylmalonic acid level and normal homocysteine level: Vitamin B_{12} or folate deficiency unlikely

- ***Anti-intrinsic Factor Antibodies / Antiparietal Cell Antibodies***

  Obtain if patient has vitamin B_{12} deficiency to assess for pernicious anemia.

  Eighty-five percent of patients with pernicious anemia have antiparietal cell antibodies (sensitive but not specific). Fifty percent of patients with pernicious anemia have anti-intrinsic factor antibodies (specific but not very sensitive).

- ***Schilling's Test***

  May help in establishing etiology of vitamin B_{12} deficiency. Consider performing if anti-intrinsic factor / antiparietal cell antibody testing is not consistent with pernicious anemia.

- ***Bone Marrow Biopsy***

  Bone marrow biopsy should be performed in the patient with macrocytic anemia and RPI <2 if the etiology is not clear and the following testing is unremarkable; liver function tests, thyroid function tests, serum folate, and serum vitamin B_{12}. It should also be obtained if the peripheral blood smear raises concern for the possibility of aplastic anemia, pure red cell aplasia, leukemia, or myelodysplastic syndrome.

MACROCYTIC ANEMIA IN THE PATIENT WITH RPI <2

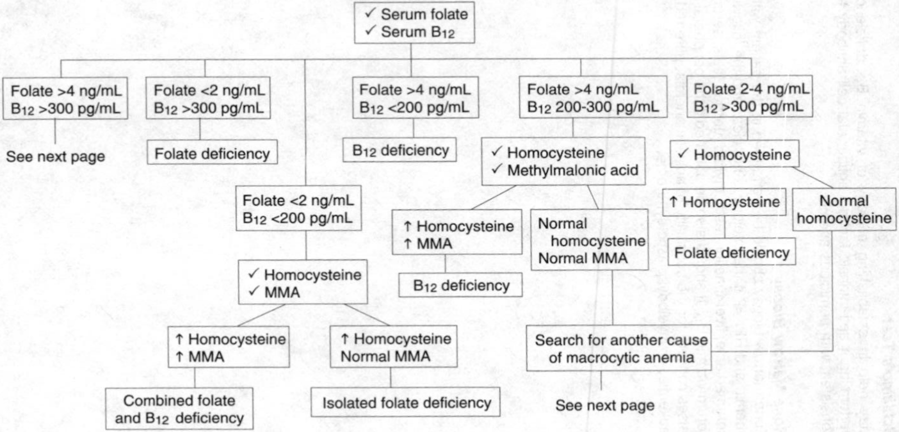
✓ Serum folate
✓ Serum B12
Folate >4 ng/mL
B12 >300 pg/mL
See next page
Folate <2 ng/mL
B12 >300 pg/mL
Folate deficiency
Folate >4 ng/mL
B12 <200 pg/mL
B12 deficiency
Folate >4 ng/mL
B12 200-300 pg/mL
✓ Homocysteine
✓ Methylmalonic acid
↑ Homocysteine
↑ MMA
B12 deficiency
Normal homocysteine
Normal MMA
Folate 2-4 ng/mL
B12 >300 pg/mL
✓ Homocysteine
↑ Homocysteine
Folate deficiency
Normal homocysteine
Search for another cause of macrocytic anemia
See next page
Folate <2 ng/mL
B12 <200 pg/mL
✓ Homocysteine
✓ MMA
↑ Homocysteine
↑ MMA
Combined folate and B12 deficiency
↑ Homocysteine
Normal MMA
Isolated folate deficiency

MMA = methylmalonic acid

MACROCYTIC ANEMIA IN THE PATIENT WITH RPI <2 *(continued)*

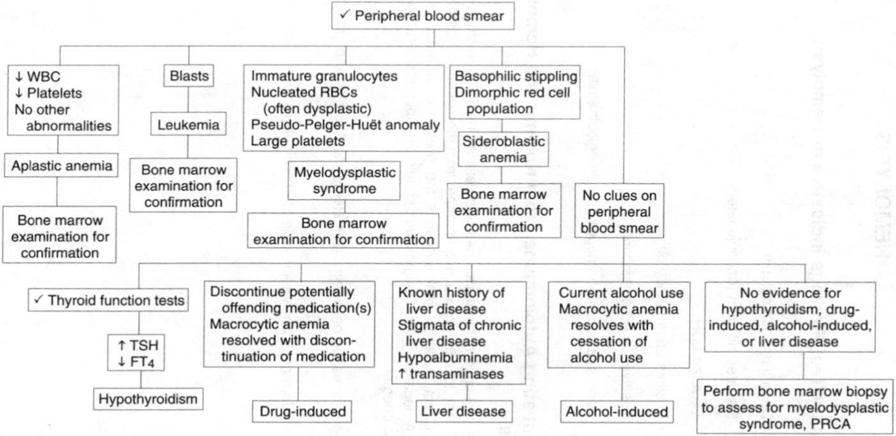
✓ Peripheral blood smear
↓ WBC
↓ Platelets
No other abnormalities
Aplastic anemia
Bone marrow examination for confirmation
Blasts
Leukemia
Bone marrow examination for confirmation
Immature granulocytes
Nucleated RBCs (often dysplastic)
Pseudo-Pelger-Huët anomaly
Large platelets
Myelodysplastic syndrome
Bone marrow examination for confirmation
Basophilic stippling
Dimorphic red cell population
Sideroblastic anemia
Bone marrow examination for confirmation
No clues on peripheral blood smear
✓ Thyroid function tests
↑ TSH
↓ FT4
Hypothyroidism
Discontinue potentially offending medication(s)
Macrocytic anemia resolved with discontinuation of medication
Drug-induced
Known history of liver disease
Stigmata of chronic liver disease
Hypoalbuminemia
↑ transaminases
Liver disease
Current alcohol use
Macrocytic anemia resolves with cessation of alcohol use
Alcohol-induced
No evidence for hypothyroidism, drug-induced, alcohol-induced, or liver disease
Perform bone marrow biopsy to assess for myelodysplastic syndrome, PRCA

HEMOLYSIS

Laboratory Test Findings Indicative of Hemolysis

- Decreased haptoglobin
- Elevated bilirubin (unconjugated)
- Elevated LDH
- Positive urine hemoglobin
- Positive urine hemosiderin
- Increased plasma hemoglobin (hemoglobinemia)

Differentiating Autoimmune From Nonimmune Hemolytic Anemia

Once the presence of hemolysis has been established, it is useful to obtain a direct Coombs' test to differentiate autoimmune from nonimmune hemolytic anemia. A positive direct Coombs' test suggests the presence of autoimmune hemolytic anemia. A negative direct Coombs' test should prompt consideration of nonimmune hemolytic anemia.

See more information on Nonimmune Hemolytic Anemia *on page 33.*

See more information on Autoimmune Hemolytic Anemia *on page 36.*

NONIMMUNE HEMOLYTIC ANEMIA

Nonimmune causes of hemolytic anemia should be considered in the patient with hemolytic anemia who has a negative direct Coombs' test.

Causes of Nonimmune Hemolytic Anemia

- Abnormalities of the red cell membrane
  - Hereditary spherocytosis
  - Hereditary elliptocytosis
  - Hereditary stomatocytosis
  - Paroxysmal nocturnal hemoglobinuria
  - Spur cell anemia
- Arsine gas
- Copper
  - Intoxication during suicide attempts
  - Wilson's disease
- Disorders within the RBC
  - Enzyme deficiency (G6PD, pyruvate kinase)
  - Hemoglobinopathies
- Hypersplenism
- Infection
  - Babesiosis
  - Bartonellosis
  - Clostridia
  - Malaria
- Microangiopathic hemolytic anemia
  - Allograft rejection
  - Disseminated intravascular coagulation
  - Disseminated cancer
  - Eclampsia
  - Hemolytic uremic syndrome
  - Malignant hypertension
  - Thrombotic thrombocytopenic purpura
- Prosthetic heart valve
- Severe burns
- Snake / spider bites

Using the Peripheral Blood Smear to Elucidate the Etiology

- *Spherocytes*: Burns, hereditary spherocytosis
- *Target cells*: Hemoglobinopathies
- *Schistocytes, helmet cells, other cell fragments*: Microangiopathic hemolytic anemia, prosthetic heart valves, severe burns
- *Bite or blister cell*: G6PD deficiency
- *Elliptocytes*: Hereditary elliptocytosis
- *Stomatocytes*: Hereditary stomatocytosis
- *Sickle cells*: Sickle cell anemia
- *Intraerythrocytic inclusions*: Malaria, babesiosis, bartonellosis
- *Heinz bodies*: G6PD deficiency

Other Laboratory Tests That May Be Indicated According to Condition Suspected

- *Hereditary spherocytosis*: Osmotic fragility test
- *Paroxysmal nocturnal hemoglobinuria*: Ham's test, sucrose hemolysis test, LAP score, cell surface markers studies (flow cytometry)
- *Spur cell anemia*: Liver function tests
- *Babesiosis*: Thick smear
- *Malaria*: Thick smear
- *G6PD deficiency*: G6PD fluorescent screening test, quantitative G6PD assay, Heinz body smear
- *Hemoglobinopathy / sickle cell anemia*: Hemoglobin electrophoresis, sodium metabisulfite test
- *Microangiopathic hemolytic anemia*: PT / PTT (for DIC), fibrinogen (for DIC), D-dimer (for DIC), BUN / creatinine (HUS or TTP), liver function tests (HELLP syndrome)

NONIMMUNE HEMOLYTIC ANEMIA

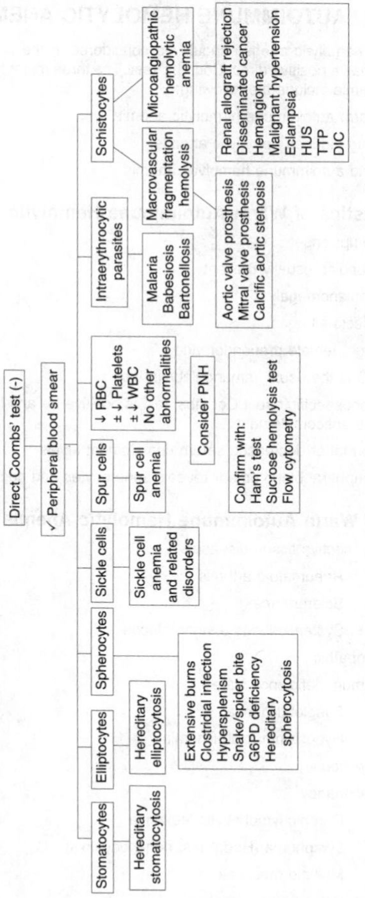
Direct Coombs' test (-)
✓ Peripheral blood smear
Stomatocytes
Hereditary stomatocytosis
Elliptocytes
Hereditary elliptocytosis
Spherocytes
Extensive burns
Clostridial infection
Hypersplenism
Snake/spider bite
G6PD deficiency
Hereditary spherocytosis
Sickle cells
Sickle cell anemia and related disorders
Spur cells
Spur cell anemia
↓ RBC
± ↓ Platelets
± ↓ WBC
No other abnormalities
Consider PNH
Confirm with:
Ham's test
Sucrose hemolysis test
Flow cytometry
Intraerythrocytic parasites
Malaria
Babesiosis
Bartonellosis
Schistocytes
Macrovascular fragmentation hemolysis
Aortic valve prosthesis
Mitral valve prosthesis
Calcific aortic stenosis
Microangiopathic hemolytic anemia
Renal allograft rejection
Disseninated cancer
Hemangioma
Malignant hypertension
Eclampsia
HUS
TTP
DIC

AUTOIMMUNE HEMOLYTIC ANEMIA

Autoimmune hemolytic anemia should be considered in the patient with hemolytic anemia who has a positive direct Coombs' test. The three major types of autoimmune hemolytic anemia include the following:

- Warm autoimmune hemolytic anemia
- Drug-induced hemolytic anemia
- Cold autoimmune hemolytic anemia

Characteristics of Warm Autoimmune Hemolytic Anemia

- Abrupt onset
- Jaundice usually present
- + splenomegaly
- Affects all ages
- Slight female preponderance
- IgG is the usual immunoglobulin type
- Monospecific direct Coombs' test is positive for anti-IgG only or anti-IgG and anticomplement
- Normal or decreased serum complement levels
- Peripheral blood smear reveals spherocytes and nucleated RBCs

Causes of Warm Autoimmune Hemolytic Anemia

- Connective tissue diseases
  - Rheumatoid arthritis
  - Scleroderma
  - Systemic lupus erythematosus
- Idiopathic
- Immunodeficiency states
  - Dysglobulinemia
  - Hypogammaglobulinemia
- Infection
- Malignancy
  - Chronic lymphocytic leukemia
  - Lymphoma (Hodgkin's, non-Hodgkin's)
  - Multiple myeloma
  - Solid tumors (rare)
  - Thymoma

Characteristics of Cold Autoimmune Hemolytic Anemia:

- Insidious onset
- Jaundice often absent
- Splenomegaly usually absent
- Affects all ages
- Predominantly affects women
- IgM is the usual immunoglobulin type
- Monospecific direct Coombs' test is positive for anticomplement only
- Decreased serum complement levels
- Peripheral blood smear reveals RBC agglutination

Causes of Cold Autoimmune Hemolytic Anemia

- Idiopathic
- Infection
  - *M. pneumoniae*
  - Epstein-Barr virus
  - CMV
- Malignancy
  - Lymphoma
  - Leukemia
  - Carcinoma
  - Myeloma

IMMUNE HEMOLYTIC ANEMIA

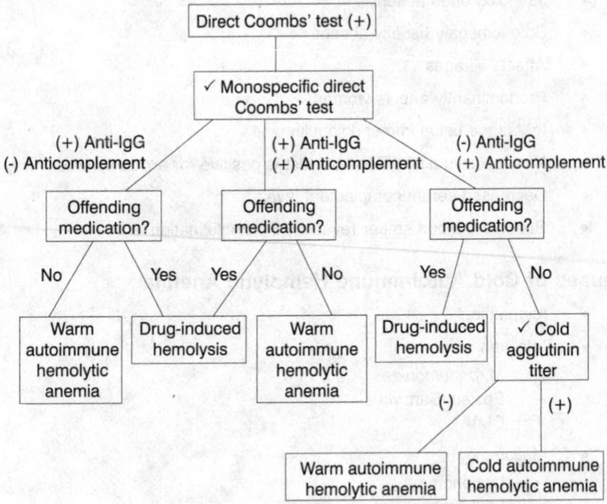
Direct Coombs' test (+)
✓ Monospecific direct Coombs' test
(+) Anti-IgG
(-) Anticomplement
(+) Anti-IgG
(+) Anticomplement
(-) Anti-IgG
(+) Anticomplement
Offending medication?
Offending medication?
Offending medication?
No
Yes
Yes
No
Yes
No
Warm autoimmune hemolytic anemia
Drug-induced hemolysis
Warm autoimmune hemolytic anemia
Drug-induced hemolysis
✓ Cold agglutinin titer
(-)
(+)
Warm autoimmune hemolytic anemia
Cold autoimmune hemolytic anemia

LEUKOCYTOSIS

White blood cells (leukocytes) include neutrophils, monocytes, lymphocytes, eosinophils, and basophils. An increase in any of these cell types can lead to leukocytosis. Leukocytosis is defined as a white blood cell count >11 x 10^9/L (11,000/mm^3).

When leukocytosis is noted, the clinician should determine which type of white blood cell is present in excess. To identify the type of white blood cell that is present in increased numbers, the clinician should examine the white blood cell differential count, which will list the percentage of each white blood cell type. These percentages are determined by an automated electronic counter or by direct examination of the peripheral blood smear.

The normal white blood cell count differential is as follows:

- Polymorphonuclear neutrophils (45% to 65%)
- Band neutrophils (0% to 5%)
- Lymphocytes (15% to 40%)
- Monocytes (2% to 8%)
- Eosinophils (0% to 5%)
- Basophils (0% to 3%)

By examining the white blood cell differential count, the clinician can categorize the leukocytosis as follows:

- Neutrophilia *on page 40*
- Lymphocytosis *on page 43*
- Eosinophilia *on page 47*
- Basophilia *on page 46*
- Monocytosis *on page 44*

NEUTROPHILIA

Neutrophilia is the most common type of leukocytosis. Neutrophilia is defined as an absolute neutrophil count that exceeds 7.5 x 10^9/L. The absolute neutrophil count is calculated by using the following formula:

ANC = total WBC count x neutrophil %

where neutrophil percentage refers to mature and band neutrophils. Band neutrophils refer to less mature neutrophils containing band-shaped nuclei.

Causes of Neutrophilia

- Infection
  - Bacterial
  - Fungal
  - Viral
  - Parasitic
  - Rickettsial
- Connective tissue disease
  - Vasculitis
  - Rheumatoid arthritis
- Malignancy
  - Stomach
  - Lung
  - Melanoma
  - Pancreatic
  - Renal
  - Hodgkin's disease
- Medications
  - Corticosteroids
  - Epinephrine
  - Lithium
  - Growth factors (G-CSF, GM-CSF)
- Myeloproliferative disorders
  - Chronic myelogenous leukemia
  - Polycythemia vera
  - Essential thrombocytosis
  - Agnogenic myeloid metaplasia
- Trauma
  - Crush injuries
  - Electric shock
  - Extremes of temperature

- Hematologic disorders
  - Hemolytic anemia
  - Recovery from marrow failure
  - Postsplenectomy
  - Myelodysplastic syndromes
  - Myelomonocytic leukemia
- Chemicals
  - Mercury poisoning
  - Ethylene glycol intoxication
  - Lead poisoning
  - Animal venom
- Metabolic conditions
  - Lactic acidosis
  - Thyrotoxicosis
  - Uremia
  - Diabetic ketoacidosis
  - Eclampsia
  - Gout
- Tissue necrosis
  - Myocardial infarction
  - Gangrene
  - Postoperative
- Physiologic neutrophilia (pseudoneutrophilia)
  - Exercise
  - Pain
  - Stress
  - Hypoxia
  - Trauma
  - Epinephrine
  - Beta-agonists
  - Seizures
  - Smoking
- Chronic idiopathic neutrophilia

NEUTROPHILIA

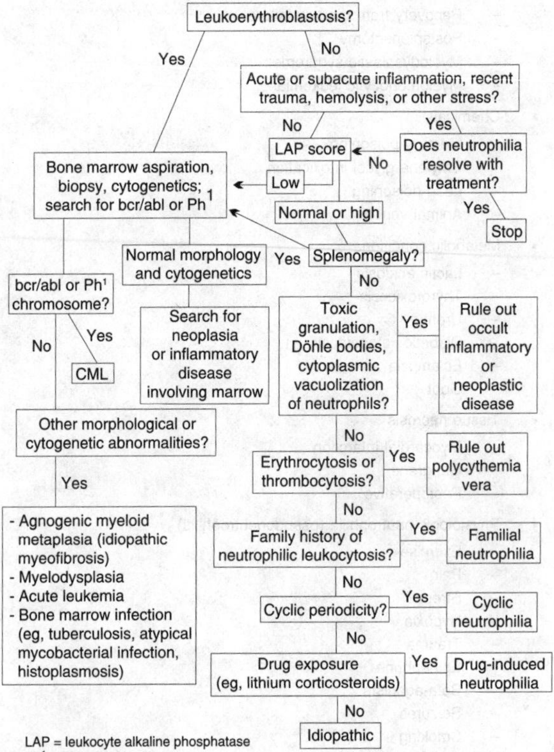
Leukoerythroblastosis?
Yes
No
Acute or subacute inflammation, recent trauma, hemolysis, or other stress?
No
Yes
LAP score
No
Does neutrophilia resolve with treatment?
Bone marrow aspiration, biopsy, cytogenetics; search for bcr/abl or Ph1
Low
Normal or high
Yes
Stop
Normal morphology and cytogenetics
Yes
Splenomegaly?
No
bcr/abl or Ph1 chromosome?
Search for neoplasia or inflammatory disease involving marrow
Toxic granulation, Döhle bodies, cytoplasmic vacuolization of neutrophils?
Yes
Rule out occult inflammatory or neoplastic disease
No
Yes
CML
Other morphological or cytogenetic abnormalities?
No
Erythrocytosis or thrombocytosis?
Yes
Rule out polycythemia vera
Yes
No
- Agnogenic myeloid metaplasia (idiopathic myeofibrosis)
- Myelodysplasia
- Acute leukemia
- Bone marrow infection (eg, tuberculosis, atypical mycobacterial infection, histoplasmosis)
Family history of neutrophilic leukocytosis?
Yes
Familial neutrophilia
No
Cyclic periodicity?
Yes
Cyclic neutrophilia
No
Drug exposure (eg, lithium corticosteroids)
Yes
Drug-induced neutrophilia
No
Idiopathic

LAP = leukocyte alkaline phosphatase
Ph1 = Philadelphia chromosome
bcr/abl = the translocation of the *c-abl* gene from chromosome 9 to the *bcr* gene on chromosome 22q
CML = chronic myelogenous leukemia

Adapted from Cecil RL, Bennett JC, and Goldman L, eds, *Cecil Textbook of Medicine*, 21st ed, Philadelphia, PA: WB Saunders Co, 1999, 931.

LYMPHOCYTOSIS

Absolute lymphocytosis is said to be present if the absolute lymphocyte count exceeds 5 x 10^9/L. The absolute lymphocyte count can be calculated as follows:

Absolute lymphocyte count = total WBC count x lymphocyte %

Causes of Lymphocytosis

- Infection
  - Viral
    - Infectious mononucleosis (Epstein-Barr virus)
    - Infectious mononucleosis-like syndrome
      - Cytomegalovirus
      - Adenovirus
      - Hepatitis (A, B, or C)
      - HIV (acute seroconversion)
      - Human herpesvirus 6
    - Other viral infection
  - Toxoplasmosis
  - Bacterial
    - Pertussis
    - Typhoid fever
    - Brucellosis
    - Tuberculosis
  - Syphilis (secondary)
  - Acute infectious lymphocytosis
- Drug reaction
- Malignancy
  - Acute lymphoblastic leukemia (early)
  - Chronic lymphocytic leukemia
  - Other chronic lymphoid leukemias
  - Hodgkin's lymphoma
  - Carcinoma
  - Thymoma
- Transient stress lymphocytosis
- Persistent polyclonal B-cell lymphocytosis
- Graves' disease
- Adrenal insufficiency

MONOCYTOSIS

Monocytosis is defined as an absolute monocyte count >0.75 x 10^9/L. The absolute monocyte count may be determined as follows:

Absolute monocyte count = total WBC count x monocyte %

Causes of Monocytosis

- Hematologic disorders
  - Leukemia
  - Lymphoma
    - Hodgkin's lymphoma
    - Non-Hodgkin's lymphoma
  - Myelodysplastic syndrome
  - Myeloproliferative disorders
  - Multiple myeloma
  - Hemolytic anemia
  - Malignant histiocytosis
  - Immune thrombocytopenic purpura
- Infection
  - Bacterial
    - Subacute bacterial endocarditis
    - Tuberculosis
    - Brucellosis
    - Typhoid fever
  - Viral
    - Infectious mononucleosis
  - Parasitic
    - Malaria
    - Leishmaniasis
  - Syphilis
  - Rickettsial (Rocky Mountain spotted fever)
- Connective tissue disease
  - Systemic lupus erythematosus
  - Rheumatoid arthritis
  - Polyarteritis nodosa

  - Temporal arteritis
  - Polymyositis
- Miscellaneous
  - Sarcoidosis
  - Splenectomy
  - Carcinoma
  - Alcoholic liver disease
  - Sprue (tropical or nontropical)
  - Inflammatory bowel disease
  - Chronic neutropenia

BASOPHILIA

Basophilia is defined as an absolute basophil count >0.2 x 10^9/L. The absolute basophil count may be determined as follows:

Absolute basophil count = total WBC count x basophil %

Causes of Basophilia

- Connective tissue disease (eg, rheumatoid arthritis)
- Ulcerative colitis
- Allergic or hypersensitivity reactions
- Endocrine disorders
  - Diabetes mellitus
  - Myxedema
- Medications
  - Antithyroid agents
  - Estrogens
- Irradiation
- Infection (eg, smallpox, chickenpox, influenza)
- Chronic renal disease
- Myeloproliferative disorders
  - Chronic myelogenous leukemia
  - Essential thrombocytosis
  - Polycythemia vera
  - Agnogenic myeloid metaplasia
- Acute myelogenous leukemia
- Carcinoma (rare)

EOSINOPHILIA

Absolute eosinophilia is said to be present if the eosinophil count is $>0.5 \times 10^9/L$. The absolute eosinophil count may be calculated using the following formula:

Absolute eosinophil count = total WBC x eosinophil %

Causes of Eosinophilia

- Infection
  - Parasitic
  - Tuberculosis
  - Scarlet fever
  - Fungal
    - Allergic bronchopulmonary aspergillosis
    - Coccidioidomycosis
- Connective tissue disease / autoimmune disorders
  - Rheumatoid arthritis
  - Polyarteritis nodosa
  - Wegener's granulomatosis
  - Churg-Strauss syndrome
  - Eosinophilic fasciitis
  - Eosinophilia-myalgia syndrome
  - Eosinophilic myositis
  - Eosinophilic gastroenteritis
  - Löffler's endocarditis
  - Ulcerative colitis
  - Regional enteritis
- Asthma
- Atopic disorders
  - Seasonal allergic rhinitis
  - Chronic urticaria
  - Atopic dermatitis
- Malignancy
  - Solid cancers
  - Hematologic
    - Acute eosinophilic leukemia

    - Chronic eosinophilic leukemia
    - T-lymphoblastic lymphoma
    - Acute lymphoblastic leukemia
    - Chronic myelogenous leukemia
    - Hodgkin's lymphoma
    - Non-Hodgkin's lymphoma

- Myelodysplastic syndrome
- Myeloproliferative disorders
- Systemic mastocytosis
- Skin diseases
  - Episodic angioedema with eosinophilia
  - Bullous pemphigoid
  - Kimura's disease
- Drug-induced
- Immunodeficiency states
- Hypereosinophilic syndrome
- Adrenal insufficiency
- Atheroembolic disease
- Eosinophilic pneumonia (acute or chronic)

NEUTROPENIA

Neutropenia is defined as an absolute neutrophil count $<1.5 \times 10^9/L$ ($1500/mm^3$). The absolute neutrophil count can be calculated by using the following formula:

Absolute neutrophil count = total WBC count x neutrophil %

where neutrophil percentage refers to mature and band neutrophils.

Causes of Neutropenia

- Infection
  - Viral
  - Bacterial
  - Fungal
  - Protozoal
  - Rickettsial
- Drug-induced
  - Dose-dependent (predictable)
  - Idiosyncratic
- Hypersplenism
- Autoimmune / other immune disorders
  - Systemic lupus erythematosus
  - Rheumatoid arthritis
  - Felty's syndrome
  - Wegener's granulomatosis
- Bone marrow replacement
  - Hematologic neoplasms
  - Solid cancer
  - Granulomatous disease
- Myelodysplastic syndrome
- Aplastic anemia
- Megaloblastic anemia (folate or B_{12} deficiency)
- Constitutional neutropenic disorders
  - Cyclic neutropenia
  - Kostmann's syndrome
  - Swachman-Diamond syndrome
  - Immunodeficiency disorders / reticular dysgenesis

  - Chédiak-Higashi syndrome
  - Myelokathexis
  - Fanconi's syndrome
  - Dyskeratosis congenital
- Acquired idiopathic neutropenia
- Irradiation

NEUTROPENIA

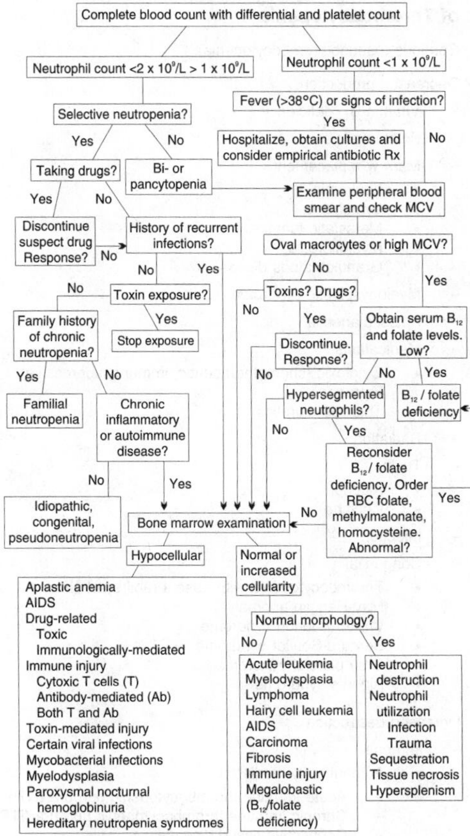
Complete blood count with differential and platelet count
Neutrophil count <2 x 10⁹/L > 1 x 10⁹/L
Neutrophil count <1 x 10⁹/L
Fever (>38°C) or signs of infection?
Yes
Hospitalize, obtain cultures and consider empirical antibiotic Rx
No
Selective neutropenia?
Yes
No
Taking drugs?
Bi- or pancytopenia
Examine peripheral blood smear and check MCV
Yes
No
Discontinue suspect drug Response?
No
History of recurrent infections?
Oval macrocytes or high MCV?
No
Yes
No
Yes
No
Toxin exposure?
Toxins? Drugs?
Yes
Family history of chronic neutropenia?
Stop exposure
No
Yes
Obtain serum B12 and folate levels. Low?
Discontinue. Response?
Yes
No
No
No
Yes
Familial neutropenia
Chronic inflammatory or autoimmune disease?
Hypersegmented neutrophils?
B12 / folate deficiency
No
Yes
Reconsider B12 / folate deficiency. Order RBC folate, methylmalonate, homocysteine. Abnormal?
No
Yes
Yes
Idiopathic, congenital, pseudoneutropenia
No
Bone marrow examination
Hypocellular
Normal or increased cellularity
Aplastic anemia
AIDS
Drug-related
Toxic
Immunologically-mediated
Immune injury
Cytoxic T cells (T)
Antibody-mediated (Ab)
Both T and Ab
Toxin-mediated injury
Certain viral infections
Mycobacterial infections
Myelodysplasia
Paroxysmal nocturnal hemoglobinuria
Hereditary neutropenia syndromes
Normal morphology?
No
Yes
Acute leukemia
Myelodysplasia
Lymphoma
Hairy cell leukemia
AIDS
Carcinoma
Fibrosis
Immune injury
Megalobastic (B12/folate deficiency)
Neutrophil destruction
Neutrophil utilization
Infection
Trauma
Sequestration
Tissue necrosis
Hypersplenism

Adapted from Goldman, Bennett, et al, *Cecil Textbook of Medicine*, 21st ed, Philadelphia, PA: WB Saunders Co, 1999, 924.

THROMBOCYTOPENIA

Causes of Thrombocytopenia

- Spurious (pseudothrombocytopenia)
- Decreased production
  - Vitamin B_{12} deficiency
  - Folate deficiency
  - Marrow replacement
    - Leukemia
    - Lymphoma
    - Metastatic tumor
    - Myelofibrosis
    - Granulomatous disease
  - Myelodysplastic syndrome
  - Aplastic anemia
  - Medications
    - Cytotoxic (chemotherapeutic, immunosuppressive)
    - Estrogens
    - Thiazide diuretics
  - Radiation
  - Toxins
    - Alcohol
    - Cocaine
  - Infection
  - Congenital
    - Thrombocytopenia with absent radii syndrome
    - May-Hegglin anomaly
    - Wiskott-Aldrich syndrome
    - Bernard-Soulier syndrome
    - Gray platelet syndrome
    - Alport's syndrome
- Increased destruction
  - Immune
    - Autoantibody-mediated
      - Acute immune thrombocytopenic purpura (ITP)
      - Chronic immune thrombocytopenic purpura (ITP)
      - Connective tissue disease
        - Systemic lupus erythematosus
        - Polyarteritis nodosa

- Malignancy
  - Chronic lymphocytic leukemia
  - Lymphoma
  - Solid tumor
- Drug-induced
- Infection (EBV, CMV, HIV, hepatitis)

- Alloantiody-mediated
  - Post-transfusion purpura
  - Neonatal

- Nonimmune
  - Hemolytic uremic syndrome (HUS)
  - Thrombotic thrombocytopenic purpura (TTP)
  - Disseminated intravascular coagulation (DIC)
  - Other causes of microangiopathic hemolytic anemia

- Hypersplenism

Risk of Bleeding

- *>100,000/μL:* No abnormal bleeding even after surgery
- *50,000-100,000/μL*: Patients may bleed longer than normal with severe trauma
- *20,000-50,000/μL:* Bleeding occurs with minor trauma
- *<20,000/μL*: Patients may have spontaneous bleeding

Peripheral Blood Smear

- *Platelet clumping or satellitism*: Consider pseudothrombocytopenia
- *Atypical lymphocytes*: Viral etiology (ie, infectious mononucleosis)
- *Fragmented red blood cells (schistocytes, helmet cells)*: Microangiopathic hemolytic anemia (HUS, TTP, DIC, etc)
- *Hypersegmented PMNs*: Megaloblastic anemia (vitamin B_{12} or folate deficiency)
- *Spherocytes + increased reticulocytes:* Evan's syndrome
- *Blasts*: Leukemia
- *Pseudo-Pelger-Huët anomaly*: Myelodysplastic syndrome
- *Leukoerythroblastosis (teardrop-shaped red blood cells, immature red blood cells, immature white blood cells)*: Myelophthisis
- *WBC left shift with Döhle bodies and cytoplasmic vacuolization*: Bacterial infection / sepsis

Other Laboratory Testing to Elucidate Etiology

- Serum folate
- Serum vitamin B_{12}
- Direct Coombs' test (if Evan's syndrome is a consideration)
- Cultures (if bacterial infection / sepsis is a consideration)
- PT / PTT (to assess for DIC if microangiopathic hemolytic anemia is present)
- D-dimer (to assess for DIC if microangiopathic hemolytic anemia is present)
- Serum BUN / creatinine (to assess for HUS or TTP if microangiopathic hemolytic anemia is present)
- Antinuclear antibodies (to assess for connective tissue disease)
- CT scan of thorax / abdomen / pelvis (to assess for lymphoma or CLL in patients who have lymphadenopathy and / or splenomegaly)
- HIV test
- Lupus anticoagulant / anticardiolipin antibodies
- Antiplatelet antibodies (can be done if ITP is suspected but testing lacks sensitivity and specificity)

Bone Marrow Biopsy

Perform if peripheral blood smear reveals blasts, features of myelodysplasia, or leukoerythroblastosis. Also perform in patients thought to have ITP if the clinical presentation is atypical or patient is >60 years of age.

THROMBOCYTOPENIA

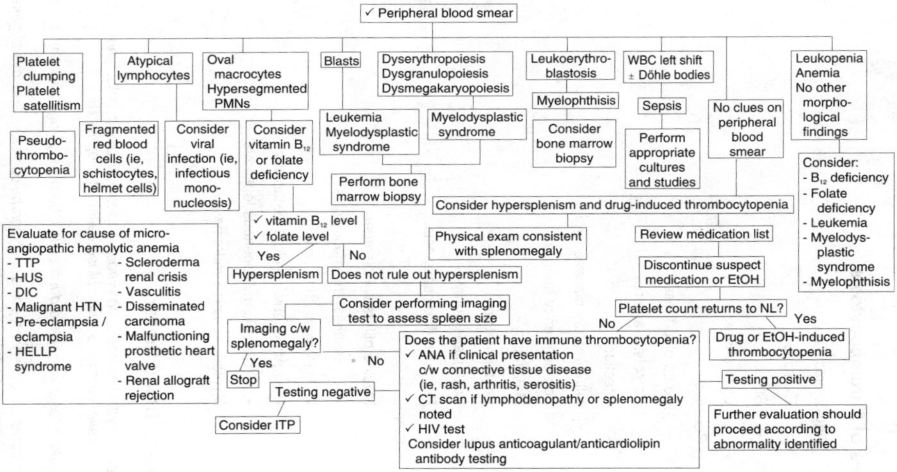
✓ Peripheral blood smear
Platelet clumping Platelet satellitism
Pseudo-thrombo-cytopenia
Fragmented red blood cells (ie, schistocytes, helmet cells)
Evaluate for cause of micro-angiopathic hemolytic anemia
- TTP
- HUS
- DIC
- Malignant HTN
- Pre-eclampsia / eclampsia
- HELLP syndrome
- Scleroderma renal crisis
- Vasculitis
- Disseminated carcinoma
- Malfunctioning prosthetic heart valve
- Renal allograft rejection
Atypical lymphocytes
Consider viral infection (ie, infectious mono-nucleosis)
Oval macrocytes Hypersegmented PMNs
Consider vitamin B_{12} or folate deficiency
✓ vitamin B_{12} level
✓ folate level
Yes
Hypersplenism
No
Does not rule out hypersplenism
Consider performing imaging test to assess spleen size
Imaging c/w splenomegaly?
Yes
Stop
No
Testing negative
Consider ITP
Blasts
Leukemia Myelodysplastic syndrome
Dyserythropoiesis Dysgranulopoiesis Dysmegakaryopoiesis
Myelodysplastic syndrome
Perform bone marrow biopsy
Leukoerythro-blastosis
Myelophthisis
Consider bone marrow biopsy
WBC left shift ± Döhle bodies
Sepsis
Perform appropriate cultures and studies
No clues on peripheral blood smear
Consider hypersplenism and drug-induced thrombocytopenia
Physical exam consistent with splenomegaly
Review medication list
Discontinue suspect medication or EtOH
Platelet count returns to NL?
Yes
Drug or EtOH-induced thrombocytopenia
No
Does the patient have immune thrombocytopenia?
✓ ANA if clinical presentation c/w connective tissue disease (ie, rash, arthritis, serositis)
✓ CT scan if lymphodenopathy or splenomegaly noted
✓ HIV test
Consider lupus anticoagulant/anticardiolipin antibody testing
Testing positive
Further evaluation should proceed according to abnormality identified
Leukopenia Anemia No other morpho-logical findings
Consider:
- B_{12} deficiency
- Folate deficiency
- Leukemia
- Myelodys-plastic syndrome
- Myelophthisis

THROMBOCYTOSIS

Causes of Thrombocytosis

- Physiologic
  - Exercise
  - Stress
  - Epinephrine
- Reactive
  - Acute blood loss
  - Hemolytic anemia
  - Infection
  - Inflammatory disease
  - Iron deficiency anemia
  - Malignancy
  - Postoperative
  - Postsplenectomy
  - Rebound thrombocytosis
- Clonal
  - Myeloproliferative disorder
    - Essential thrombocytosis
    - Polycythemia vera
    - Agnogenic myeloid metaplasia
    - Chronic myelogenous leukemia
  - Myelodysplastic syndrome

Peripheral Blood Smear

Leukoerythroblastosis (teardrop-shaped red blood cells, immature red blood cells, immature white blood cells): Myelophthisis

Leukocytosis with marked left shift: Chronic myelogenous leukemia

Features of dyserythropoiesis, dysgranulopoiesis, and dysmegakaryopoiesis: Myelodysplastic syndrome

Other Laboratory Tests to Elucidate Etiology

- Serum ferritin
- C-reactive protein; elevated level suggests reactive thrombocytosis
- Elevated hemoglobin; consider myeloproliferative disorder
- Red cell mass (if polycythemia vera is a consideration)

Bone Marrow Biopsy

- Perform if reactive cause of thrombocytosis not present
- Cytogenetic testing should be performed to assess for Philadelphia chromosome found in CML
- Significant fibrosis supports diagnosis of agnogenic myeloid metaplasia

THROMBOCYTOSIS

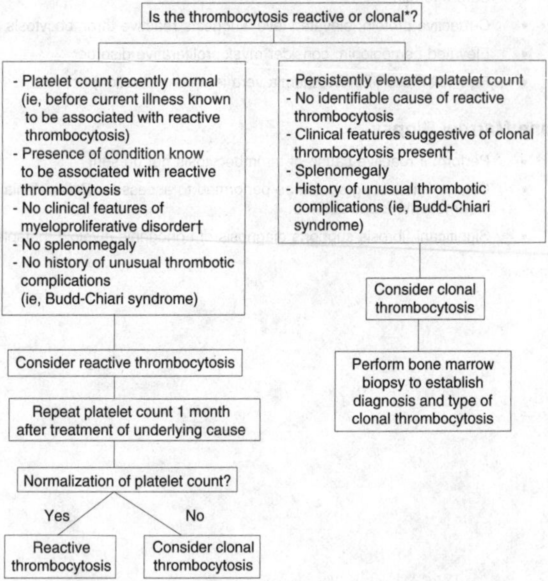
Is the thrombocytosis reactive or clonal*?
- Platelet count recently normal (ie, before current illness known to be associated with reactive thrombocytosis)
- Presence of condition know to be associated with reactive thrombocytosis
- No clinical features of myeloproliferative disorder†
- No splenomegaly
- No history of unusual thrombotic complications (ie, Budd-Chiari syndrome)
- Persistently elevated platelet count
- No identifiable cause of reactive thrombocytosis
- Clinical features suggestive of clonal thrombocytosis present†
- Splenomegaly
- History of unusual thrombotic complications (ie, Budd-Chiari syndrome)
Consider clonal thrombocytosis
Perform bone marrow biopsy to establish diagnosis and type of clonal thrombocytosis
Consider reactive thrombocytosis
Repeat platelet count 1 month after treatment of underlying cause
Normalization of platelet count?
Yes
No
Reactive thrombocytosis
Consider clonal thrombocytosis

*Clonal thrombocytosis occurs in patients with myeloproliferative disorders or myelodysplastic syndrome. Myeloproliferative disorders include essential thrombocytosis, CML, PCV, and agnogenic myeloid metaplasia.

†The presence of postbathing pruritus should prompt consideration of PCV. Erythromelalgia, which refers to painful, red, ischemic digits, may occur in patients with PCV or essential thrombocytosis. Striking pelthora may be noted in some PCV patients.

ELEVATED PT (NORMAL PTT)

Note: The following discussion is pertinent to the patient with an isolated prolongation of the PT (normal PTT).

Causes of Elevated PT (Normal PTT)

- Common
  - Liver disease (early)
  - Coumadin® therapy
  - Vitamin K deficiency (early)
- Uncommon
  - Factor VII deficiency
  - Factor VII inhibitor
  - Lupus anticoagulant

Establishing the Etiology

- Elevated PT due to coumadin therapy is usually apparent.
- Factor VII deficiency or inhibitor is rare.
- Mixing study is useful in elucidating the etiology. In this study, equal parts of the patient's plasma are mixed with plasma derived from a pool of normal donors. This will result in correction of the PT if the elevated PT is due to a deficiency of one or more factors. There will be little to no correction of the PT if an inhibitory antibody is present.
- In usual clinical practice (if the patient is not on coumadin therapy), causes of ↑ PT include liver disease and vitamin K deficiency.
- In patients with PT elevation due to liver disease, the etiology is usually apparent after consideration of the patient's symptoms, signs, laboratory testing, and imaging test results. Some patients with liver disease, however, may also have vitamin K deficiency.
- Vitamin K deficiency may be the result of inadequate intake, antibiotic therapy, or malabsorption (or combination thereof).
- To differentiate between vitamin K deficiency and liver disease, it is useful to assess the response to vitamin K administration.
  - Return of PT back to normal range = vitamin K deficiency
  - No decrease in the PT = liver disease
  - Some decrease in the PT but not to within normal range = liver disease + vitamin K deficiency

↑PT (Normal PTT)

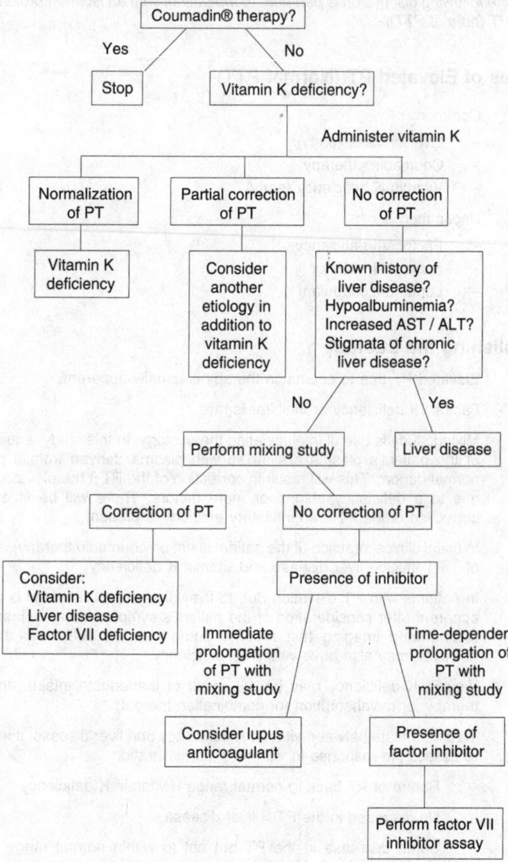
Coumadin® therapy?
Yes
No
Stop
Vitamin K deficiency?
Administer vitamin K
Normalization of PT
Partial correction of PT
No correction of PT
Vitamin K deficiency
Consider another etiology in addition to vitamin K deficiency
Known history of liver disease? Hypoalbuminemia? Increased AST / ALT? Stigmata of chronic liver disease?
No
Yes
Perform mixing study
Liver disease
Correction of PT
No correction of PT
Consider: Vitamin K deficiency Liver disease Factor VII deficiency
Presence of inhibitor
Immediate prolongation of PT with mixing study
Time-dependent prolongation of PT with mixing study
Consider lupus anticoagulant
Presence of factor inhibitor
Perform factor VII inhibitor assay

ELEVATED PTT (NORMAL PT)

Note: The following discussion is pertinent to the patient with an isolated prolongation of the PTT (normal PT).

Causes of Elevated PTT (Normal PT)

- Heparin therapy
- Factor deficiency (VIII, IX, XI, XII, high molecular weight kininogen, prekallikrein)
- von Willebrand's disease
- Factor inhibitor (to VIII, IX, XI, XII, high molecular weight kininogen, prekallikrein)
- Lupus anticoagulant

Establishing the Etiology

- Elevated PTT due to heparin therapy is usually apparent.
- Mixing study is useful in elucidating the etiology. In this study, equal parts of patient's plasma are mixed with plasma derived from a pool of normal donors. This will result in correction of the PTT if the elevated PTT is due to a deficiency of one or more factors. There will be little to no correction of the PTT if an inhibitory antibody is present.
- If the PTT corrects with the mixing study, the focus should be on factor deficiencies:
  - If there is a history of bleeding disorder, consider deficiency of factor VIII (hemophilia A), IX (hemophilia B), XI, or von Willebrand's disease.
  - If there is no history of bleeding disorder, consider deficiency of XII, high molecular weight kininogen, or prekallikrein.
  - Specific factor assays need to be performed to establish the diagnosis. If von Willebrand's disease is suspected, factor VIII activity, ristocetin cofactor activity, and vWF antigen tests should be performed. If these tests are suggestive of the diagnosis, further testing may include ristocetin-induced platelet agglutination and vWF multimeric analysis to identify the subtype of von Willebrand's disease that is present.

  If the PTT does not correct with the mixing study, the focus should be on an inhibitor (factor inhibitor or lupus anticoagulant):
  - To differentiate between factor inhibitor and the lupus anticoagulant, the results of the mixing study should be examined carefully. The mixing study involves assessment of the PTT immediately, as well as 1-2 hours after the addition of normal plasma. Lupus anticoagulant

characteristically results in immediate prolongation of the PTT with a similar value obtained 1-2 hours later. In contrast, factor inhibitors show time-dependent prolongation (progressive prolongation of the PTT over 1-2 hours).

- Factor VIII inhibitors develop not only in patients with hemophilia A but also with advancing age, during pregnancy/postpartum period, and in patients with connective tissue disease (SLE, rheumatoid arthritis).
- Factor IX inhibitors may develop in patients with hemophilia B.
- The presence of the lupus anticoagulant is established when the following criteria are met:
  1. Prolonged PTT, dilute Russell viper venom test (dRVVT), or kaolin clotting time (KCT)
  2. Failure of the above clotting tests to correct with the addition of normal plasma (mixing study)
  3. Normalization of the above clotting abnormalities with the use of frozen platelets (platelet neutralization procedure)
- If lupus anticoagulant testing is positive, the clinician should evaluate the patient for the antiphospholipid syndrome. Other tests that should be obtained include anticardiolipin antibodies, antibodies against β_2-glycoprotein I, and serologic test for syphilis.

↑ PTT (Normal PT)

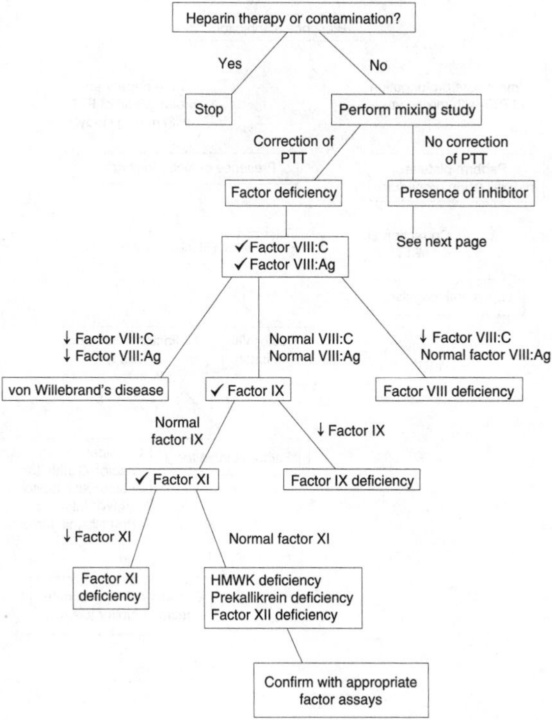
Heparin therapy or contamination?
Yes
No
Stop
Perform mixing study
Correction of PTT
No correction of PTT
Factor deficiency
Presence of inhibitor
See next page
✓Factor VIII:C
✓Factor VIII:Ag
↓ Factor VIII:C
↓ Factor VIII:Ag
Normal VIII:C
Normal VIII:Ag
↓ Factor VIII:C
Normal factor VIII:Ag
von Willebrand's disease
✓ Factor IX
Factor VIII deficiency
Normal factor IX
↓ Factor IX
✓ Factor XI
Factor IX deficiency
↓ Factor XI
Normal factor XI
Factor XI deficiency
HMWK deficiency
Prekallikrein deficiency
Factor XII deficiency
Confirm with appropriate factor assays

↑ PTT (Normal PT) *(continued)*

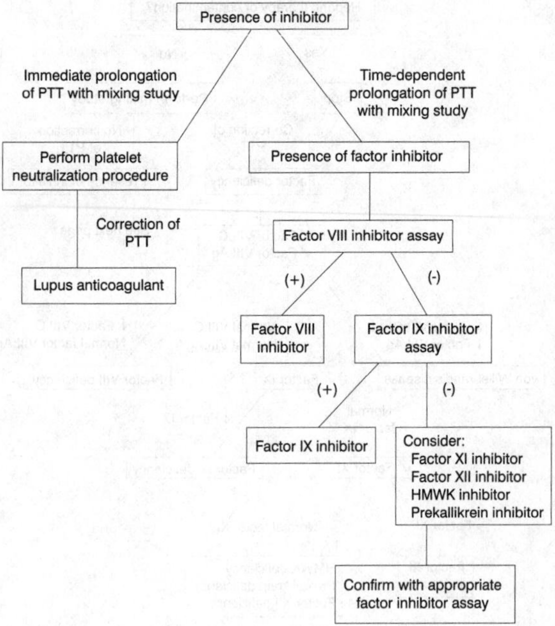
Presence of inhibitor
Immediate prolongation of PTT with mixing study
Time-dependent prolongation of PTT with mixing study
Perform platelet neutralization procedure
Presence of factor inhibitor
Correction of PTT
Factor VIII inhibitor assay
Lupus anticoagulant
(+)
(-)
Factor VIII inhibitor
Factor IX inhibitor assay
(+)
(-)
Factor IX inhibitor
Consider:
Factor XI inhibitor
Factor XII inhibitor
HMWK inhibitor
Prekallikrein inhibitor
Confirm with appropriate factor inhibitor assay

ELEVATED PT AND PTT

Causes of Elevated PT and PTT

- Common pathway factor deficiencies (I, II, V, X)
- Heparin
- Coumadin® therapy
- Vitamin K deficiency
- Liver disease
- Disseminated intravascular coagulation (DIC)
- Lupus anticoagulant
- Factor inhibitor (to I, II, V, X)
- Primary fibrinolysis
- Dysfibrinogenemia

Establishing the Etiology

- If DIC is suspected, initial laboratory testing should include platelet count, coagulation times (PT, PTT), fibrinogen level, peripheral blood smear, and D-dimer. The classic laboratory test findings seen in DIC include:
  - Thrombocytopenia
  - Elevated PT and PTT
  - Decreased fibrinogen
  - Schistocytes on peripheral blood smear
  - Elevated D-dimer

  This picture is more likely to be seen with acute DIC. In chronic DIC, lab test results are more variable. The best test is the D-dimer. Without an increased D-dimer, it is difficult to make the diagnosis of DIC.
- Liver disease should be suspected when symptoms, signs, liver function test abnormalities, and imaging test results consistent with severe liver disease are present. To differentiate liver disease from DIC, one useful test is the factor VIII level, which is normal or increased in liver disease but decreased in DIC.
- Early vitamin K deficiency may present with only an isolated prolongation of the PT but as the severity of the deficiency worsens, the PTT will rise as well. Resolution of the coagulation abnormalities with vitamin K replacement establishes the diagnosis.
- Heparin therapy is typically associated with an isolated elevation of the PTT but with excessive doses, the PT will rise as well.

- Coumadin therapy is typically associated with an isolated elevation of the PT but with excessive doses, the PTT will rise as well.
- Mixing study is useful in elucidating the etiology. In this study, equal parts of patient's plasma are mixed with plasma derived from a pool of normal donors. This will result in correction of the PT/PTT if the elevated PT/PTT is due to a deficiency of one or more factors. There will be little to no correction of the PT/PTT if an inhibitory antibody is present.
  - If the PT/PTT corrects with the mixing study, the focus should be on deficiency of one or more factors (see causes above).
  - If the PT/PTT does not correct with the mixing study, the focus should be on the presence of an inhibitor (factor inhibitor or lupus anticoagulant).

↑ PT / ↑ PTT

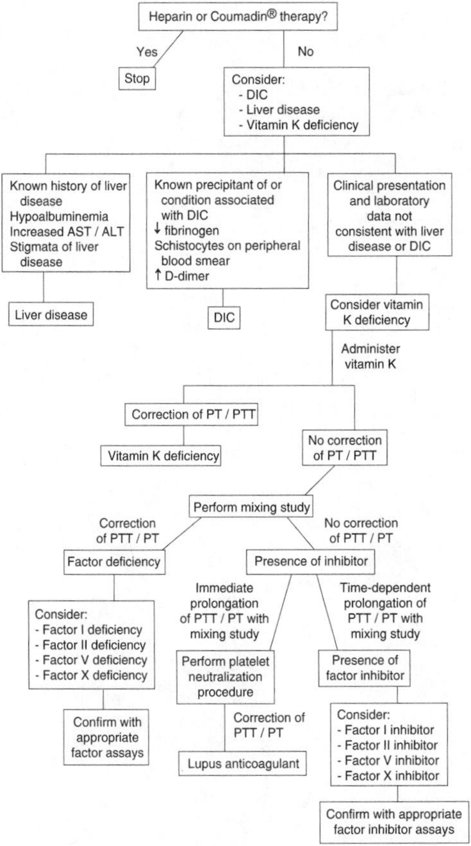
Heparin or Coumadin® therapy?
Yes
Stop
No
Consider:
- DIC
- Liver disease
- Vitamin K deficiency
Known history of liver disease
Hypoalbuminemia
Increased AST / ALT
Stigmata of liver disease
Liver disease
Known precipitant of or condition associated with DIC
↓ fibrinogen
Schistocytes on peripheral blood smear
↑ D-dimer
DIC
Clinical presentation and laboratory data not consistent with liver disease or DIC
Consider vitamin K deficiency
Administer vitamin K
Correction of PT / PTT
Vitamin K deficiency
No correction of PT / PTT
Perform mixing study
Correction of PTT / PT
Factor deficiency
Consider:
- Factor I deficiency
- Factor II deficiency
- Factor V deficiency
- Factor X deficiency
Confirm with appropriate factor assays
No correction of PTT / PT
Presence of inhibitor
Immediate prolongation of PTT / PT with mixing study
Perform platelet neutralization procedure
Correction of PTT / PT
Lupus anticoagulant
Time-dependent prolongation of PTT / PT with mixing study
Presence of factor inhibitor
Consider:
- Factor I inhibitor
- Factor II inhibitor
- Factor V inhibitor
- Factor X inhibitor
Confirm with appropriate factor inhibitor assays

FLUIDS, ELECTROLYTES, & ACID BASE

HYPONATREMIA

Causes of Hyponatremia

- Spurious hyponatremia
  - "Drip-arm" hyponatremia
  - "Dead-space" hyponatremia
- Isotonic hyponatremia
  - Pseudohyponatremia (hyperlipidemia, hyperproteinemia)
- Hypertonic hyponatremia
  - Hyperglycemia
  - Mannitol administration
  - Glycine
  - Maltose
- Hypotonic hyponatremia
  - Hypovolemic
    - Extrarenal
      - Gastrointestinal fluid loss (vomiting, diarrhea, blood loss)
      - Skin losses of fluid (excessive sweating)
      - Third-space fluid loss (bowel obstruction, pancreatitis, peritonitis, burns, muscle trauma)
    - Renal
      - Salt-losing nephropathies
      - Diuretic therapy
      - Osmotic diuresis (glucose, urea, mannitol)
      - Mineralocorticoid deficiency
      - Ketonuria
      - Bicarbonaturia
      - Cerebral salt-wasting syndrome
  - Euvolemic
    - Syndrome of inappropriate antidiuretic hormone (SIADH)
    - Adrenal insufficiency

- Hypothyroidism
- Thiazide diuretics
- Primary polydipsia
- Decreased intake of solutes (beer drinkers' potomania, tea-and-toast diet)

– Hypervolemic
- Congestive heart failure
- Cirrhosis
- Nephrotic syndrome
- Acute renal failure
- Chronic renal failure

Establishing the Etiology

- Initial step is to measure the plasma osmolality which will help place the patient into one of the following categories:
  – Hypotonic hyponatremia (plasma osmolality <280 mOsm/kg)
  – Isotonic hyponatremia (plasma osmolality between 280-295 mOsm/kg)
  – Hypertonic hyponatremia (plasma osmolality >295 mOsm/kg)
- Hypertonic hyponatremia may be seen in patients with significant hyperglycemia or with the administration of hypertonic mannitol
- Isotonic hyponatremia should prompt consideration of hyperproteinemia or hyperlipidemia
- Most patients will have hypotonic hyponatremia. The initial evaluation involves assessment of the patient's volume status. Based upon the volume status, patients can be categorized into one of the three groups, as shown in the following table.

PHYSICAL EXAM FINDINGS USED TO ASSESS VOLUME STATUS

Finding in Physical Examination	Volume Status
Orthostatic changes in blood pressure and heart rate Dry mucous membranes Poor skin turgor Flat jugular veins Absence of axillary sweat	Hypovolemic
Peripheral edema Elevated jugular venous pressure Ascites Other signs of congestive heart failure, cirrhosis, or nephrotic syndrome	Hypervolemic
Absence of physical exam findings consistent with hypervolemia or hypovolemia	Euvolemic

- Approach to the patient with hypovolemic hypotonic hyponatremia
  - The causes of hypovolemic hypotonic hyponatremia can be divided into renal and extrarenal causes (see causes above).
  - The cause is usually evident after a thorough history and physical examination.
  - If the etiology is unclear, a urine sodium level may be obtained. Urine sodium level <20 mEq/L should prompt consideration of an extrarenal cause while a level >20 mEq/L is suggestive of a renal etiology.
- Approach to the patient with hypervolemic hypotonic hyponatremia
  - Causes of hypervolemic hypotonic hyponatremia include congestive heart failure, cirrhosis, nephrotic syndrome, and renal failure (acute or chronic).
  - Etiology is usually readily apparent after a thorough history and physical examination.
  - If the etiology is unclear, a urine sodium level may be obtained. Urine sodium level <20 mEq/L is consistent with congestive heart failure, cirrhosis, and nephrotic syndrome. A level exceeding 20 mEq/L is suggestive of acute or chronic renal failure.
- Approach to the patient with euvolemic hypotonic hyponatremia
  - Causes of euvolemic hypotonic hyponatremia include SIADH, hypothyroidism, adrenal insufficiency, thiazide diuretics, primary polydipsia, or decreased intake of solutes (beer drinkers' potomania).
  - Urine osmolality is useful in narrowing the differential diagnosis further. Urine osmolality <100 mOsm/kg is consistent with primary polydipsia or beer drinkers' potomania. The other causes are associated with a urine osmolality >100 mOsm/kg.
  - Criteria for SIADH, the most common cause of this type of hyponatremia are listed in the following box.

ESSENTIAL CRITERIA FOR SIADH

Normal acid-base balance	Inappropriate urinary concentration (urine osmolality >100 mOsm/kg)
Normal adrenal function	Euvolemic volume status
Normal renal function	Urine sodium >40 mEq/L
Normal thyroid function	
Plasma osmolality <270 mOsm/kg	

  - In order to truly satisfy the diagnosis of SIADH, hypothyroidism and adrenal insufficiency must be excluded by performing thyroid function tests and the cosyntropin stimulation test, respectively.

– If SIADH is diagnosed, every effort should be made to identify the etiology. The causes of SIADH are listed in the following box.

SIADH DIFFERENTIAL DIAGNOSIS

LUNG DISEASE
- Abscess
- Chronic obstructive pulmonary disease
- Pneumonia (viral, bacterial)
- Tuberculosis
- Aspergillosis
- Acute bronchial asthma
- Bronchiectasis
- Empyema
- Cystic fibrosis
- Pneumothorax

CNS CONDITIONS
- Brain tumor
- Cerebrovascular accident
- Encephalitis
- Meningitis
- Subarachnoid hemorrhage
- Subdural hematoma
- Acute psychosis
- Head trauma
- Brain abscess
- Cavernous sinus thrombosis
- Multiple sclerosis
- Acute intermittent porphyria
- Guillan-Barré syndrome
- Delirium tremens
- Hydrocephalus

POSITIVE PRESSURE VENTILATION

STRESS / PAIN

MEDICATIONS
- Chlorpropamide
- Cyclophosphamide
- Opiates
- Tegretol
- Tricyclic antidepressants
- Vincristine / Vinblastine
- SSRIs
- Oxytocin
- Ifosfamide
- Desmopressin
- Lysine vasopressin
- Clofibrate
- Prostaglandin synthesis inhibitors
- Nicotine
- Antipsychotics
- Acetaminophen
- NSAIDs

MALIGNANCY
- Lymphoma
- Pancreatic cancer
- Small cell cancer of lung
- Pharyngeal carcinoma
- Duodenal cancer
- Thymoma
- Mesothelioma
- Bladder carcinoma
- Prostate cancer
- Reticulum cell sarcoma
- Ureteric cancer
- Endometrial cancer

MDMA / ECSTASY

MISCELLANEOUS
- Postoperative state
- Severe nausea
- HIV infection

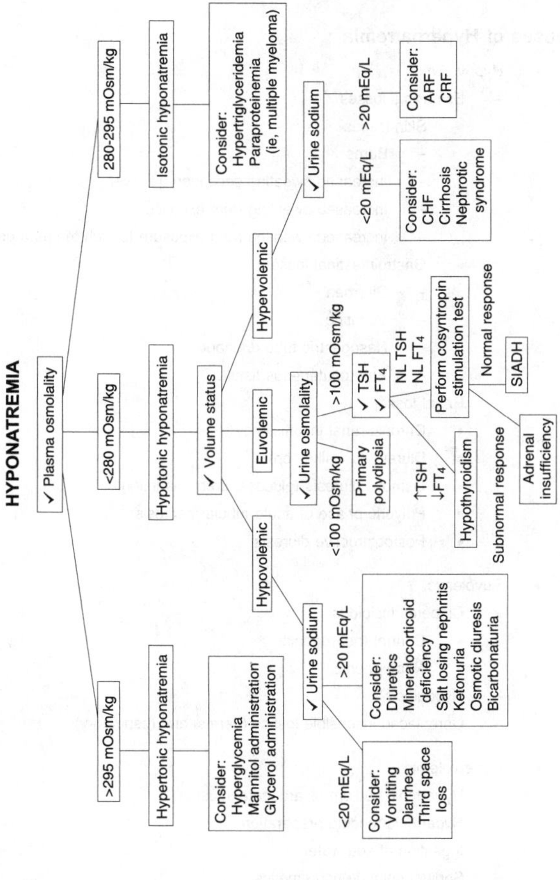
HYPONATREMIA
✓ Plasma osmolality
>295 mOsm/kg
<280 mOsm/kg
280-295 mOsm/kg
Hypertonic hyponatremia
Hypotonic hyponatremia
Isotonic hyponatremia
Consider: Hyperglycemia Mannitol administration Glycerol administration
✓ Volume status
Consider: Hypertriglyceridemia Paraproteinemia (ie, multiple myeloma)
Hypovolemic
Euvolemic
Hypervolemic
✓ Urine sodium
✓ Urine osmolality
✓ Urine sodium
<20 mEq/L
>20 mEq/L
<100 mOsm/kg
>100 mOsm/kg
<20 mEq/L
>20 mEq/L
Consider: Vomiting Diarrhea Third space loss
Consider: Diuretics Mineralocorticoid deficiency Salt losing nephritis Ketonuria Osmotic diuresis Bicarbonaturia
Primary polydipsia
✓ TSH ✓ FT4
Consider: CHF Cirrhosis Nephrotic syndrome
Consider: ARF CRF
↑TSH ↓FT4
NL TSH NL FT4
Hypothyroidism
Perform cosyntropin stimulation test
Subnormal response
Normal response
Adrenal insufficiency
SIADH

HYPERNATREMIA

Causes of Hypernatremia

- Hypovolemic
  - Extrarenal losses
    - Skin losses
      - Burns
      - Increased sweating secondary to fever
      - Increased sweating from exercise
      - Increased sweating from exposure to high temperatures
    - Gastrointestinal losses
      - Diarrhea
      - Vomiting
      - Nasogastric tube drainage
      - Enterocutaneous fistula
  - Renal losses
    - Chronic renal insufficiency
    - Diuretic (usually loop)
    - Osmotic diuresis (glucose, urea, mannitol)
    - Polyuric phase of acute tubular necrosis
    - Postobstructive diuresis

- Euvolemic
  - Diabetes insipidus
    - Central (neurogenic)
    - Nephrogenic
  - Hypodipsia
  - Unreplaced insensible losses (dermal and respiratory)

- Hypervolemic
  - Hypertonic sodium bicarbonate infusion
  - Hypertonic feeding preparation
  - Ingestion of sea water
  - Sodium chloride-rich emetics

- Ingestion of sodium chloride
- Hypertonic sodium chloride infusion
- Hypertonic dialysis
- Hypertonic saline enemas
- Cushing's syndrome
- Primary hyperaldosteronism

Establishing the Etiology

- The cause of the hypernatremia is usually apparent after a thorough history and physical examination.
- If the etiology is not clear, an assessment of the volume status will allow the patient to be categorized into one of the following groups:

PHYSICAL EXAM FINDINGS USED TO ASSESS VOLUME STATUS

Findings in the Physical Exam	Volume Status
Orthostatic changes in blood pressure and heart rate Dry mucous membranes Poor skin turgor Flat jugular veins Absence of axillary sweat	Hypovolemic
Peripheral edema Elevated jugular venous pressure	Hypervolemic
No findings consistent with hypervolemia or hypovolemia	Euvolemic

- Approach to the patient with hypovolemic hypernatremia
  - Etiology of hypovolemic hypernatremia is usually apparent after a thorough history and physical examination.
  - Causes of hypovolemic hypernatremia can be divided into extrarenal and renal causes (see causes above).
  - A urine sodium level is often helpful in differentiating between renal and extrarenal causes of hypovolemic hypernatremia. Urine sodium level <20 mEq/L should prompt consideration of an extrarenal cause while a level >20 mEq/L is more suggestive of a renal etiology.

- The urine osmolality level is also helpful in differentiating between renal and extrarenal causes. Urine osmolality >700 mOsm/kg should prompt consideration of an extrarenal cause. In renal causes, the urine is less than maximally concentrated.

- Etiology of hypervolemic hypernatremia is readily apparent (see causes above).

- Approach to the patient with euvolemic hypernatremia
  - Main causes of euvolemic hypernatremia are diabetes insipidus and unreplaced insensible losses (dermal and respiratory).
  - The urine osmolality is helpful in differentiating between these two possibilities. Urine osmolality >700 mOsm/kg is suggestive of unreplaced insensible losses whereas a level <700 mOsm/kg should prompt consideration of diabetes insipidus.
  - Diabetes insipidus may be central (defect in secretion of ADH) or nephrogenic (defect in the action of ADH at the level of the kidney). In patients with diabetes insipidus, the water deprivation test can be used to differentiate between central and nephrogenic causes. The causes of diabetes insipidus are listed below.

CAUSES OF CENTRAL (NEUROGENIC) DIABETES INSIPIDUS	
GRANULOMATOUS DISEASE	POST-TRAUMATIC
Histiocytosis	CYSTS
Sarcoidosis	CEREBROVASCULAR DISEASE
Wegener's granulomatosis	Hypoxic or ischemic encephalopathy
Tuberculosis	(cardiopulmonary arrest, shock,
IDIOPATHIC	Sheehan's syndrome)
INFECTION	Aneurysm
Encephalitis	Cerebrovascular accident
Meningitis	Cavernous sinus thrombosis
Syphilis	MALIGNANCY
Tuberculosis	Craniopharyngioma
Toxoplasmosis	Leukemia
MISCELLANEOUS	Metastatic cancer (breast, lung)
Anorexia nervosa	Lymphoma
Guillan-Barré syndrome	Pinealoma
PITUITARY SURGERY	Pituitary tumor

The causes of nephrogenic diabetes insipidus are listed in the following box.

CAUSES OF NEPHROGENIC DIABETES INSIPIDUS

CONGENITAL

ACQUIRED

Medications

Amphotericin B	Foscarnet	Ethacrynic acid
Demeclocycline	Ifosfamide	Phenytoin
Lithium	Propoxyphene (overdose)	Acetohexamide
Methoxyflurane	Colchicine	Tolazamide
Streptozotocin	Gentamicin	Glyburide
Vasopressin	Methicillin	Norepinephrine
V_2-receptor antagonist	Furosemide	Vinblastine

Electrolyte disorders

Hypercalcemia	Hypokalemia

Renal disease

Obstructive uropathy	Sickle cell nephropathy	Sarcoidosis
Medullary cystic disease	Analgesic nephropathy	Polycystic kidney disease
Sjögren's syndrome	Systemic lupus erythematosus	Multiple myeloma
Amyloidosis		

HYPERNATREMIA

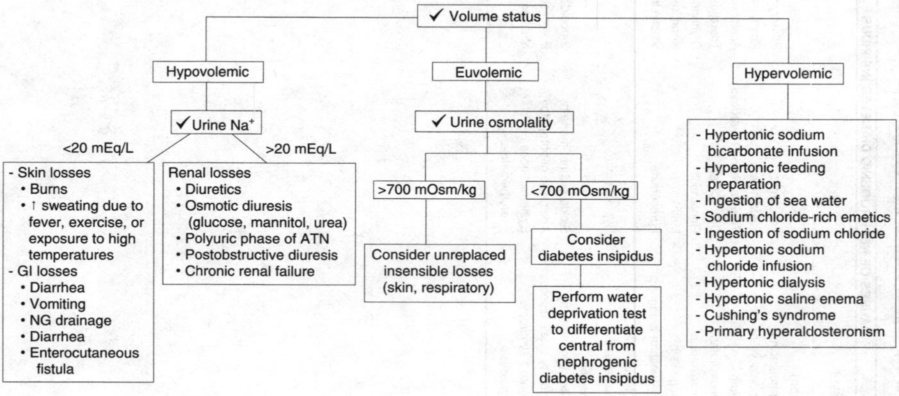
✓ Volume status
Hypovolemic
Euvolemic
Hypervolemic
✓ Urine Na+
<20 mEq/L
>20 mEq/L
- Skin losses
• Burns
• ↑ sweating due to fever, exercise, or exposure to high temperatures
- GI losses
• Diarrhea
• Vomiting
• NG drainage
• Diarrhea
• Enterocutaneous fistula
Renal losses
• Diuretics
• Osmotic diuresis (glucose, mannitol, urea)
• Polyuric phase of ATN
• Postobstructive diuresis
• Chronic renal failure
✓ Urine osmolality
>700 mOsm/kg
<700 mOsm/kg
Consider unreplaced insensible losses (skin, respiratory)
Consider diabetes insipidus
Perform water deprivation test to differentiate central from nephrogenic diabetes insipidus
- Hypertonic sodium bicarbonate infusion
- Hypertonic feeding preparation
- Ingestion of sea water
- Sodium chloride-rich emetics
- Ingestion of sodium chloride
- Hypertonic sodium chloride infusion
- Hypertonic dialysis
- Hypertonic saline enema
- Cushing's syndrome
- Primary hyperaldosteronism

HYPOKALEMIA

Causes of Hypokalemia

- Pseudohypokalemia
- Decreased potassium intake
- Redistribution
  - Alkalemia
  - Insulin administration
  - β_2-adrenergic agonist
  - Anabolic states
    - Therapy of pernicious anemia
    - Growth factor therapy
    - Rapidly growing leukemias / lymphomas
    - Response to total parenteral nutrition
    - Refeeding syndrome
  - Hypokalemic periodic paralysis
  - Theophylline overdose
  - Barium salt poisoning
  - Increased endogenous catecholamine release
    - Myocardial infarction
    - Delirium tremens
    - Head trauma
    - Cardiac surgery
    - Other stressful illnesses
  - Hypothermia
  - Multiple transfusions of frozen, washed RBCs
  - Acute chloroquine intoxication
- Excess potassium loss
  - Gastrointestinal (vomiting, diarrhea, fistula)
  - Skin (excessive exercise in hot climates, extensive burns)
  - Renal - associated with hypertension
    - Malignant hypertension
    - Renin-secreting tumor
    - Renovascular hypertension

  - Glucocorticoid suppressible aldosteronism
  - Primary hyperaldosteronism
  - Congenital adrenal hyperplasia
  - Cushing's syndrome
  - 11-β-hydroxysteroid dehydrogenase inhibition
  - Syndrome of apparent mineralocorticoid excess
  - Liddle's syndrome
  - Diuretic therapy
- Renal - not associated with hypertension
  - Renal tubular acidosis
    - Proximal (type II)
    - Distal (type I)
  - Diuretic therapy
  - Bartter's syndrome
  - Gitelman's syndrome
  - Vomiting / nasogastric drainage
  - Antibiotic use
    - Penicillin
    - Amphotericin B
    - Aminoglycosides
  - Hypomagnesemia
  - Lysozymuria

Establishing the Etiology

- Cause of hypokalemia is often readily apparent after a thorough history and physical examination (see causes above)
- If the etiology is unclear, consider the possibility of spurious hypokalemia, decreased potassium intake, gastrointestinal loss of potassium, or redistribution:
  - Spurious hypokalemia (pseudohypokalemia) may be seen with markedly elevated WBC counts.
  - Decreased potassium intake is a rare cause of hypokalemia but may be a contributing factor, often exacerbating hypokalemia due to other causes.
  - The causes of hypokalemia secondary to redistribution are listed above (see causes above).
  - Gastrointestinal loss of potassium (ie, diarrhea) is usually apparent.

- If spurious hypokalemia, decreased potassium intake, gastrointestinal loss of potassium, or redistribution are unlikely to be the cause of the hypokalemia, the clinician should assess the urine potassium level. The urine potassium level is helpful in narrowing the differential diagnosis of hypokalemia:
  - Spot urine specimen or 24-hour urine collection for potassium may be obtained but 24-hour urine collection is probably more accurate.
  - A 24-hour urine potassium >25-30 mEq/day is consistent with a condition causing renal loss of potassium whereas a level below this should prompt consideration of an extrarenal cause.
  - A spot urine potassium >15-20 mEq/L is consistent with a condition causing renal loss of potassium whereas a level below this should prompt consideration of an extrarenal cause.
- If a condition causing renal loss of potassium is present, the next step is to assess the patient's blood pressure and acid-base status:
  - In the normotensive patient, the acid-base status is helpful in narrowing the differential diagnosis, as shown in the following table.

USING THE ACID-BASE STATUS TO DETERMINE THE ETIOLOGY OF HYPOKALEMIA IN THE NORMOTENSIVE PATIENT WITH RENAL LOSSES OF POTASSIUM

Blood Pressure	Acid-Base Status	Conditions Suggested
Normal	Metabolic acidosis	Proximal RTA Distal RTA Toluene exposure
Normal	Metabolic alkalosis	Bartter's syndrome Gitelman's syndrome Diuretic use Vomiting
Normal	Normal	Antibiotic (high dose of penicillin, carbenicillin, oxacillin, ampicillin) Cisplatin therapy Hypomagnesemia Lysozymuria

  - In the hypertensive patient with hypokalemia, the etiology is often evident from the history and physical examination. If the etiology is unclear, the clinical presentation and measurement of the plasma renin activity (PRA) and aldosterone may help (see algorithm) identify which one of the following causes is present:

HYPOKALEMIA AND HYPERTENSION DIFFERENTIAL DIAGNOSIS

Malignant hypertension
Renin-secreting tumors
Renovascular hypertension
Glucocorticoid suppressible aldosteronism
Primary hyperaldosteronism
Congenital adrenal hyperplasia
Cushing's syndrome
11-β-hydroxysteroid dehydrogenase inhibition
Liddle's syndrome
Diuretic therapy
Syndrome of apparent mineralocorticoid excess

HYPOKALEMIA

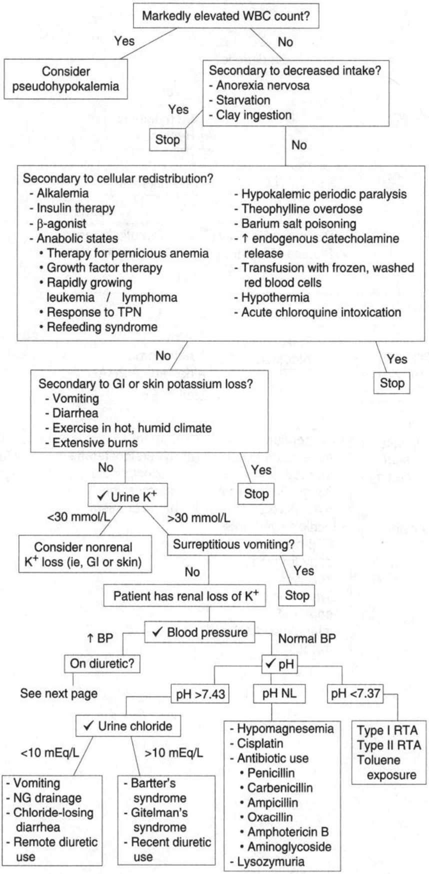
Markedly elevated WBC count?
Yes
No
Consider pseudohypokalemia
Secondary to decreased intake?
- Anorexia nervosa
- Starvation
- Clay ingestion
Yes
Stop
No
Secondary to cellular redistribution?
- Alkalemia
- Insulin therapy
- β-agonist
- Anabolic states
• Therapy for pernicious anemia
• Growth factor therapy
• Rapidly growing leukemia / lymphoma
• Response to TPN
• Refeeding syndrome
- Hypokalemic periodic paralysis
- Theophylline overdose
- Barium salt poisoning
- ↑ endogenous catecholamine release
- Transfusion with frozen, washed red blood cells
- Hypothermia
- Acute chloroquine intoxication
No
Yes
Stop
Secondary to GI or skin potassium loss?
- Vomiting
- Diarrhea
- Exercise in hot, humid climate
- Extensive burns
No
Yes
Stop
✓ Urine K+
<30 mmol/L
>30 mmol/L
Consider nonrenal K+ loss (ie, GI or skin)
Surreptitious vomiting?
No
Yes
Stop
Patient has renal loss of K+
✓ Blood pressure
↑ BP
Normal BP
On diuretic?
See next page
✓ pH
pH >7.43
pH NL
pH <7.37
✓ Urine chloride
<10 mEq/L
>10 mEq/L
- Vomiting
- NG drainage
- Chloride-losing diarrhea
- Remote diuretic use
- Bartter's syndrome
- Gitelman's syndrome
- Recent diuretic use
- Hypomagnesemia
- Cisplatin
- Antibiotic use
• Penicillin
• Carbenicillin
• Ampicillin
• Oxacillin
• Amphotericin B
• Aminoglycoside
- Lysozymuria
Type I RTA
Type II RTA
Toluene exposure

HYPOKALEMIA (*continued*)

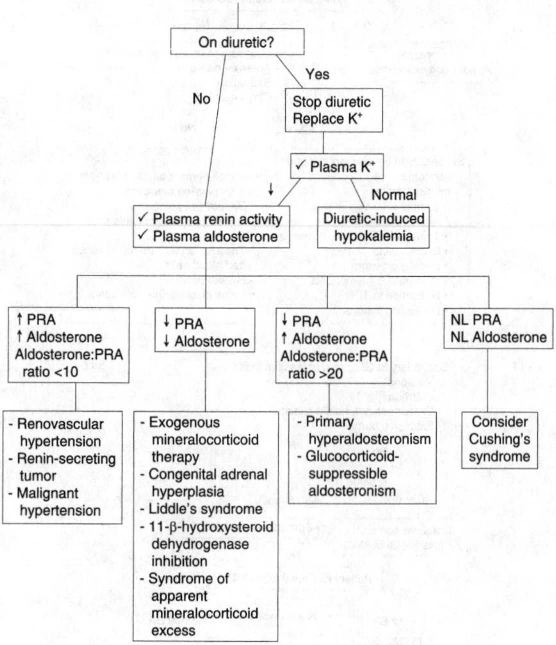
On diuretic?
Yes
No
Stop diuretic
Replace K+
✓ Plasma K+
↓
Normal
✓ Plasma renin activity
✓ Plasma aldosterone
Diuretic-induced hypokalemia
↑ PRA
↑ Aldosterone
Aldosterone:PRA ratio <10
↓ PRA
↓ Aldosterone
↓ PRA
↑ Aldosterone
Aldosterone:PRA ratio >20
NL PRA
NL Aldosterone
- Renovascular hypertension
- Renin-secreting tumor
- Malignant hypertension
- Exogenous mineralocorticoid therapy
- Congenital adrenal hyperplasia
- Liddle's syndrome
- 11-β-hydroxysteroid dehydrogenase inhibition
- Syndrome of apparent mineralocorticoid excess
- Primary hyperaldosteronism
- Glucocorticoid-suppressible aldosteronism
Consider Cushing's syndrome

HYPERKALEMIA

Causes of Hyperkalemia

- Pseudohyperkalemia
- Increased potassium intake
- Redistribution
  - Metabolic acidosis
  - Insulin deficiency
  - Hyperosmolality
  - Succinylcholine
  - Arginine hydrochloride
  - Somatostatin
  - Hyperkalemic periodic paralysis
  - β_2-receptor blocker
  - Tissue catabolism
  - Digoxin overdose
  - Severe exercise
  - Cardiac surgery
- Decreased urinary excretion
  - Renal failure (acute or chronic)
  - Hypoaldosteronism
    - Hyporeninemic hypoaldosteronism
    - Gordon's syndrome
    - Adrenal insufficiency
    - Congenital adrenal hyperplasia
    - Medications
      - Heparin
      - Cyclosporine
      - ACE inhibitors
      - Angiotensin II receptor antagonists
      - NSAIDs
  - Aldosterone resistance

- Potassium-sparing diuretics
  - Spironolactone
  - Triamterene
  - Amiloride
- Trimethoprim
- Pentamidine
- Renal tubular disorders
  - Systemic lupus erythematosus
  - Obstructive uropathy
  - Amyloidosis
  - Renal transplant
  - Sickle cell disease
  - Medullary cystic disease
  - Lead nephropathy
  - Idiopathic interstitial nephritis

Establishing the Etiology

- Consider the possibility of spurious hyperkalemia (pseudohyperkalemia):
  - May occur with repeated vigorous fist clenching, *in vitro* cell lysis (hemolysis), lysis of platelets in patients with marked thrombocytosis, or lysis of white blood cells in patients with marked leukocytosis.
  - If suspected, make every effort to obtain specimen carefully and correctly (brief use of tourniquet, avoid repeat clenching of fist, use heparinized specimen, separate plasma from cells within an hour of the venipuncture).
  - No further evaluation necessary if repeat potassium level is normal.
- Consider the possibility of hyperkalemia due to redistribution:
  - Refers to the movement of potassium from the intracellular to extracellular fluid.
  - The causes of hyperkalemia due to redistribution are listed above.
- Consider the possibility of hyperkalemia due to increased intake of potassium:
  - Unusual for increased intake of potassium to be the sole cause of hyperkalemia.
  - Not unusual for increased intake of potassium to be a contributing factor, especially in patients who have a condition that impairs the urinary excretion of potassium.

- Consider the possibility of hyperkalemia due to decreased urinary excretion of potassium:
  - Causes of hyperkalemia due to decreased urinary excretion of potassium are listed above.
  - Acute and chronic renal failure may both cause hyperkalemia. In chronic renal failure, hyperkalemia is uncommon unless the GFR <10-15 mL/minute.
  - Careful medication history will reveal medication-induced hyperkalemia (ACE inhibitor, potassium-sparing diuretic, NSAIDs, heparin, trimethoprim, pentamidine, and cyclosporine).
  - Adrenal insufficiency should be considered, especially in patients with symptoms of weakness, fatigue, nausea, vomiting, anorexia, abdominal pain, diarrhea, constipation, and weight loss. Orthostatic hypotension and hyperpigmentation are some physical exam findings of adrenal insufficiency. If suspected, a cosyntropin stimulation test should be performed.
  - Hyporeninemic hypoaldosteronism should be considered, especially if typical features are present. Typical features include older age, mild to moderate chronic renal insufficiency (creatinine clearance 15-70 mL/minute), and diabetes mellitus (present in about 50% of patients).

HYPERKALEMIA

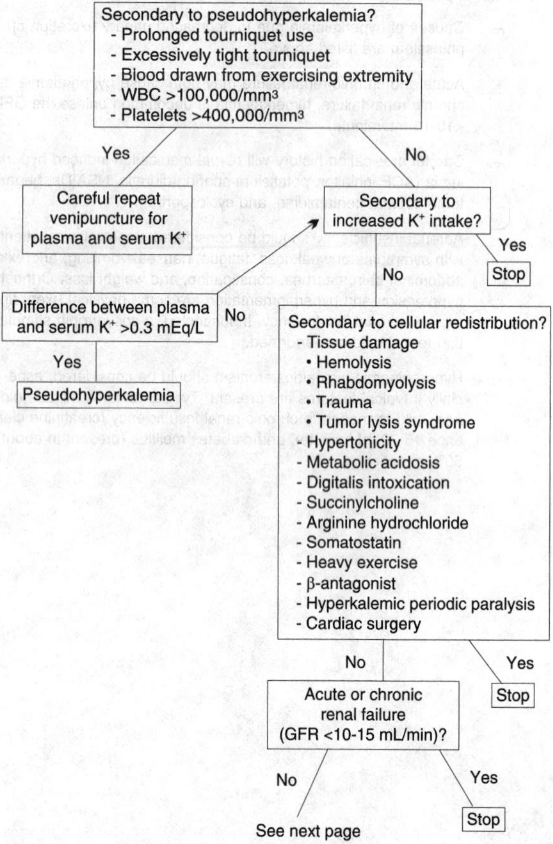
Secondary to pseudohyperkalemia?
- Prolonged tourniquet use
- Excessively tight tourniquet
- Blood drawn from exercising extremity
- WBC >100,000/mm3
- Platelets >400,000/mm3
Yes
No
Careful repeat venipuncture for plasma and serum K+
Secondary to increased K+ intake?
Yes
Stop
No
Difference between plasma and serum K+ >0.3 mEq/L
No
Yes
Pseudohyperkalemia
Secondary to cellular redistribution?
- Tissue damage
• Hemolysis
• Rhabdomyolysis
• Trauma
• Tumor lysis syndrome
- Hypertonicity
- Metabolic acidosis
- Digitalis intoxication
- Succinylcholine
- Arginine hydrochloride
- Somatostatin
- Heavy exercise
- β-antagonist
- Hyperkalemic periodic paralysis
- Cardiac surgery
No
Yes
Stop
Acute or chronic renal failure (GFR <10-15 mL/min)?
No
Yes
Stop
See next page

HYPERKALEMIA *(continued)*

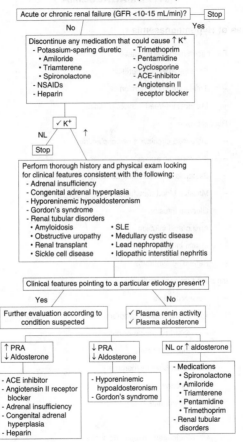

Acute or chronic renal failure (GFR <10-15 mL/min)?

- Yes → Stop
- No ↓

Discontinue any medication that could cause ↑ K^+

- Potassium-sparing diuretic
  - Amiloride
  - Triamterene
  - Spironolactone
- NSAIDs
- Heparin
- Trimethoprim
- Pentamidine
- Cyclosporine
- ACE-inhibitor
- Angiotensin II receptor blocker

↓

✓ K^+

- NL → Stop
- ↑ ↓

Perform thorough history and physical exam looking for clinical features consistent with the following:

- Adrenal insufficiency
- Congenital adrenal hyperplasia
- Hyporeninemic hypoaldosteronism
- Gordon's syndrome
- Renal tubular disorders
  - Amyloidosis
  - Obstructive uropathy
  - Renal transplant
  - Sickle cell disease
  - SLE
  - Medullary cystic disease
  - Lead nephropathy
  - Idiopathic interstitial nephritis

↓

Clinical features pointing to a particular etiology present?

- Yes → Further evaluation according to condition suspected
- No → ✓ Plasma renin activity; ✓ Plasma aldosterone

↑ PRA, ↓ Aldosterone

- ACE inhibitor
- Angiotensin II receptor blocker
- Adrenal insufficiency
- Congenital adrenal hyperplasia
- Heparin

↓ PRA, ↓ Aldosterone

- Hyporeninemic hypoaldosteronism
- Gordon's syndrome

NL or ↑ aldosterone

- Medications
  - Spironolactone
  - Amiloride
  - Triamterene
  - Pentamidine
  - Trimethoprim
- Renal tubular disorders

HYPOMAGNESEMIA

Causes of Hypomagnesemia

- Decreased magnesium intake
  - Protein-calorie malnutrition
  - Total parenteral nutrition
  - Magnesium-free intravenous fluids
- Redistribution
  - Increased circulating catecholamines
  - β-adrenergic agonists
  - Systemic acidosis (after correction)
  - Massive blood transfusion
  - Glucose infusion
  - Amino acid infusion
  - Insulin infusion
  - Refeeding syndrome
- Increased magnesium loss
  - Gastrointestinal
    - Malabsorption syndromes
    - Diarrhea (acute or chronic)
    - Intestinal fistula
    - Short bowel syndrome
    - Laxative abuse
    - Pancreatitis
    - Emesis
    - Prolonged nasogastric suction
    - Primary intestinal hypomagnesemia

- Renal
    - Medications
        - Diuretics (loop, thiazide, osmotic)
        - Cisplatin
        - Aminoglycosides
        - Pentamidine
        - Cyclosporine A
        - Tacrolimus
        - Amphotericin B
    - Acute tubular necrosis (recovery or diuretic phase)
    - Volume expansion
    - Alcoholism / alcohol withdrawal
    - Diabetes mellitus
    - Endocrine disorders
        - Hyperparathyroidism
        - Hyperthyroidism
        - Hyperaldosteronism (primary or secondary)
        - Inappropriate ADH secretion
        - Hypercalcemia
    - Postrenal transplantation
    - Postobstructive diuresis
    - Genetic conditions
        - Bartter's syndrome
        - Gitelman's syndrome
        - Primary renal magnesium wasting
    - Phosphate depletion
- Miscellaneous
    - Severe burns
    - Cardiopulmonary bypass
    - Excessive sweating
    - Excessive lactation
    - Last trimester of pregnancy
    - Foscarnet
    - Hypoalbuminemia

HYPERMAGNESEMIA

Causes of Hypermagnesemia

- Increased intake
  - Magnesium-containing cathartics
  - Magnesium-containing antacids
  - Rectal administration of magnesium salts
  - Magnesium sulfate infusion (eclampsia)
  - Urethral irrigation with hemiacidrin
  - Swallowing sea water during near-drowning in Dead Sea
- Renal failure
  - Acute renal failure (oliguric phase)
  - Chronic renal failure
- Adrenal insufficiency
- Familial hypocalciuric hypercalcemia
- Primary hyperparathyroidism
- Tumor lysis syndrome
- Milk-alkali syndrome
- Dehydration
- Acute acidosis

HYPOCALCEMIA

Causes of Hypocalcemia

- Hypoparathyroidism
- PTH resistance
  - Pseudohypoparathyroidism
  - Hypomagnesemia
- Vitamin D deficiency
- 1-α-hydroxylase deficiency (vitamin D-dependent rickets type I)
- Vitamin D resistance (vitamin D-dependent rickets type II)
- Malignancy
  - Osteoblastic metastases
  - Tumor lysis syndrome
- Sepsis
- Hungry bone syndrome
- Rhabdomyolysis
- Medications
  - Plicamycin
  - Calcitonin
  - Bisphosphonates
  - Phosphate
  - Phenobarbital
  - Citrated blood
  - Radiographic contrast dyes
  - Fluoride
  - Foscarnet
  - Pentamidine
- Acute pancreatitis
- Toxic shock syndrome

Establishing the Etiology

- In patients with hypoalbuminemia, add 0.8 mg/dL to the total serum calcium concentration for every 1 g/dL the serum albumin is <4 g/dL.
  - If the total serum calcium corrects to within the normal range, no further evaluation is necessary.
  - If the total serum calcium does not correct to within the normal range, further evaluation is necessary.
- The serum phosphate level may provide clues to the etiology of the hypocalcemia.
  - Elevated serum phosphate levels should prompt consideration of hypoparathyroidism, pseudohypoparathyroidism, or acute/chronic renal failure.
  - Low or normal serum phosphate levels should prompt consideration of vitamin D deficiency, decreased 25-hydroxyvitamin D generation (liver disease, anticonvulsants), vitamin D-dependent rickets type I/II, acute pancreatitis, or hypomagnesemia.
  - Although the serum phosphate level may provide a clue to the etiology of the hypocalcemia, the level may be affected by many factors. For this reason, further evaluation is usually necessary to establish the etiology of the hypocalcemia.
- In many cases of hypocalcemia, the patient's clinical presentation is such that the cause is readily apparent (acute pancreatitis, sepsis, medications, hungry bone syndrome, tumor lysis syndrome, osteoblastic metastases, rhabdomyolysis, chronic renal failure, hypomagnesemia).
- If the cause is not readily apparent, serum PTH level should be obtained
  - Low serum PTH level should prompt consideration of primary hypoparathyroidism or hypomagnesemia
  - High serum PTH level should prompt consideration of the following:
    1. Vitamin D deficiency
    2. Vitamin D-dependent rickets type I/II
    3. Pseudohypoparathyroidism
    4. Severe liver disease
    5. Chronic renal failure
    6. Nephrotic syndrome
  - Clinical presentation and appropriate testing usually allow the clinician to differentiate among the above conditions (see table on next page).

BIOCHEMICAL FINDINGS IN HYPOCALCEMIC CONDITIONS ASSOCIATED WITH INCREASED PTH

Diagnosis	Phosphate	PTH	25(OH)D	$1,25(OH)_2D3$
Vitamin D deficiency	↓	↑	↓	↓, NL, ↑
Severe liver disease	↓	↑	↓	↓, NL, ↑
Chronic renal failure	↑	↑	NL	↓
Nephrotic syndrome	↓	↑	↓	↓, NL
Pseudo- hypoparathyroidism	↑	↑	NL	↓
Vitamin D-dependent rickets type I	↓	↑	NL, ↑	↓
Vitamin D-dependent rickets type II	↓	↑	NL, ↑	↑

HYPOCALCEMIA

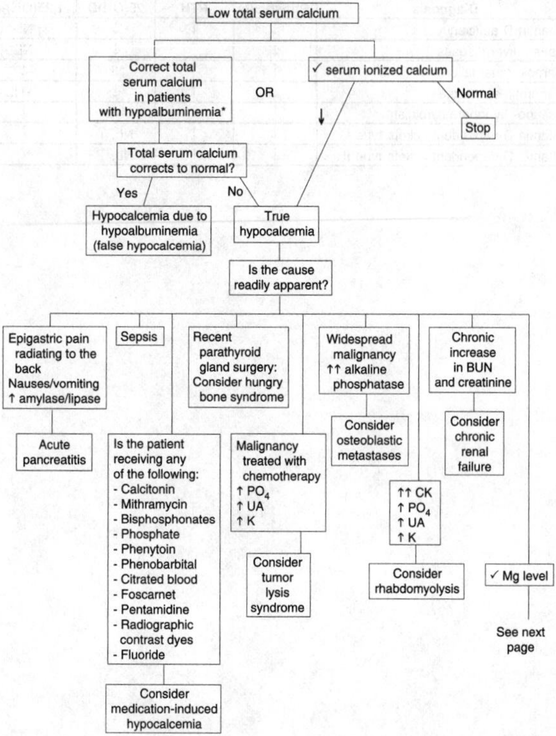
Low total serum calcium
Correct total serum calcium in patients with hypoalbuminemia*
OR
✓ serum ionized calcium
Normal
Stop
↓
Total serum calcium corrects to normal?
Yes
No
Hypocalcemia due to hypoalbuminemia (false hypocalcemia)
True hypocalcemia
Is the cause readily apparent?
Epigastric pain radiating to the back
Nauses/vomiting
↑ amylase/lipase
Acute pancreatitis
Sepsis
Is the patient receiving any of the following:
- Calcitonin
- Mithramycin
- Bisphosphonates
- Phosphate
- Phenytoin
- Phenobarbital
- Citrated blood
- Foscarnet
- Pentamidine
- Radiographic contrast dyes
- Fluoride
Consider medication-induced hypocalcemia
Recent parathyroid gland surgery: Consider hungry bone syndrome
Malignancy treated with chemotherapy
↑ PO4
↑ UA
↑ K
Consider tumor lysis syndrome
Widespread malignancy
↑↑ alkaline phosphatase
Consider osteoblastic metastases
↑↑ CK
↑ PO4
↑ UA
↑ K
Consider rhabdomyolysis
Chronic increase in BUN and creatinine
Consider chronic renal failure
✓ Mg level
See next page

*Corrected calcium = measured calcium + 0.8 (4 - patient's albumin)

HYPOCALCEMIA *(continued)*

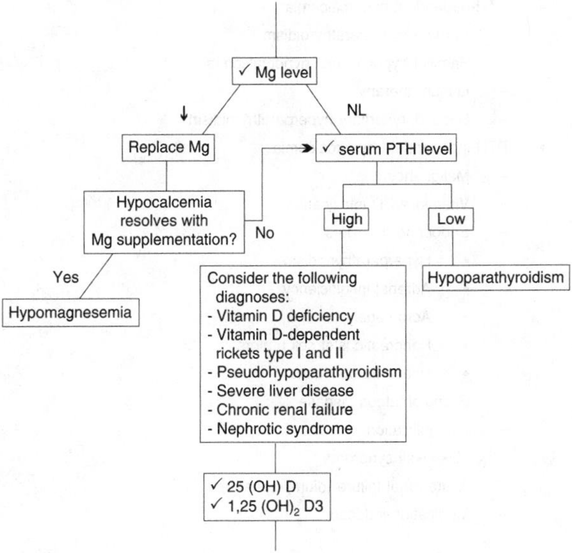
✓ Mg level
↓
NL
Replace Mg
✓ serum PTH level
Hypocalcemia resolves with Mg supplementation?
No
High
Low
Yes
Consider the following diagnoses:
- Vitamin D deficiency
- Vitamin D-dependent rickets type I and II
- Pseudohypoparathyroidism
- Severe liver disease
- Chronic renal failure
- Nephrotic syndrome
Hypoparathyroidism
Hypomagnesemia
✓ 25 (OH) D
✓ 1,25 $(OH)_2$ D3

See table "Biochemical Findings in Hypocalcemic Conditions Associated With Increased PTH," on page 95.

HYPERCALCEMIA

Causes of Hypercalcemia

- PTH-dependent hypercalcemia
  - Primary hyperparathyroidism
  - Familial hypocalciuric hypercalcemia
  - Lithium therapy
  - Secondary/tertiary hyperparathyroidism
- PTH-independent hypercalcemia
  - Malignancy
  - Vitamin A / D intoxication
  - Endocrine disorders
    - Hyperparathyroidism
    - Adrenal insufficiency
    - Acromegaly
    - Pancreatic islet cell tumors
    - Pheochromocytoma
  - Granulomatous disease
  - Immobilization
  - Milk-alkali syndrome
  - Acute renal failure (diuretic phase)
  - Medication-induced

Establishing the Etiology

- In patients with hypoalbuminemia, add 0.8 mg/dL to the total serum calcium concentration for every 1 g/dL the serum albumin is <4 g/dL. This is important because some patients with hypercalcemia may be missed if this correction is not made.
- The two major causes of hypercalcemia, accounting for 80% to 90% of cases, are primary hyperparathyroidism and malignancy.
- The serum PTH level should be obtained in the hypercalcemic patient:
  - An elevated serum PTH level should prompt consideration of primary hyperparathyroidism, lithium therapy, tertiary hyperparathyroidism, and familial hypocalciuric hypercalcemia.
  - All other causes of hypercalcemia will usually present with low serum PTH levels.

- In patients who have high serum PTH levels, the etiology is usually primary hyperparathyroidism:
  - Lithium therapy should be considered, however, if the patient is on such therapy.
  - Tertiary hyperparathyroidism typically occurs in end-stage renal disease patient.
  - Familial hypocalciuric hypercalcemia needs to be distinguished from primary hyperparathyroidism. Features favoring a diagnosis of the former include asymptomatic hypercalcemia and urinary calcium to creatinine clearance <0.01.
- In patients with low serum PTH levels, the initial focus should be on malignancy:
  - Most patients will have known cancer but, in some, hypercalcemia, may be the initial manifestation of an underlying neoplasm; most of these patients will have signs and symptoms of an undiagnosed malignancy.
  - Hypercalcemia that has persisted for >6 months is unlikely to be malignancy-related because most of these patients succumb to their disease within months.
- If malignancy is not the cause, other causes of hypercalcemia presenting with low serum PTH levels should be considered:
  - If vitamin D intoxication suspected, obtain 25-hydroxyvitamin D level.
  - If the triad of hypercalcemia, alkalosis, and renal insufficiency is present, consider milk alkali syndrome.
  - If the patient has granulomatous disease, obtain 1,25 dihydroxyvitamin D level to support the diagnosis of hypercalcemia due to granulomatous disease.
  - If hyperthyroidism suspected, obtain thyroid function tests.
  - Review medication list for thiazide diuretic, theophylline, or antiestrogen use.
  - Consider also vitamin A intoxication, immobilization, adrenal insufficiency, acromegaly, pheochromocytoma, islet cell tumors of pancreas, diuretic phase of acute renal failure, and total parenteral nutrition.

HYPERCALCEMIA

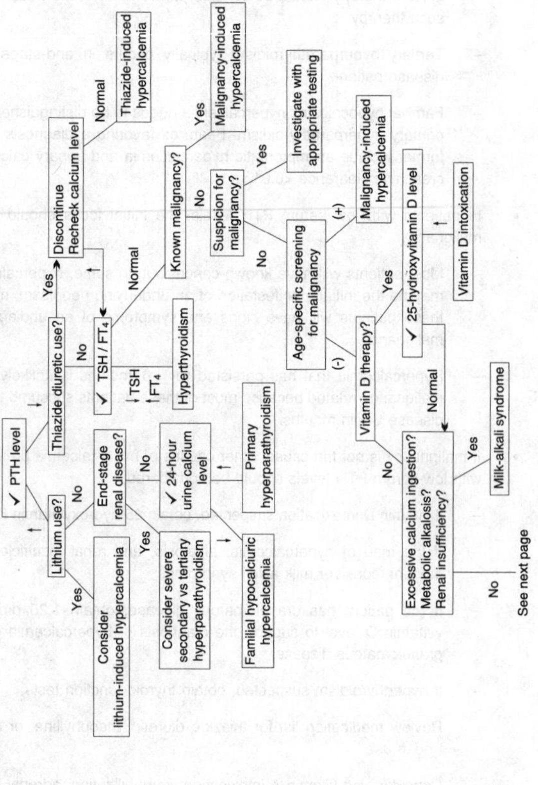
✓ PTH level
Lithium use?
Thiazide diuretic use?
Yes
No
Consider lithium-induced hypercalcemia
End-stage renal disease?
Yes
Discontinue
Recheck calcium level
Normal
Thiazide-induced hypercalcemia
✓ TSH / FT4
Consider severe secondary vs tertiary hyperparathyroidism
✓ 24-hour urine calcium level
TSH
FT4
Hyperthyroidism
Known malignancy?
Malignancy-induced hypercalcemia
Suspicion for malignancy?
Investigate with appropriate testing
Familial hypocalciuric hypercalcemia
Primary hyperparathyroidism
Age-specific screening for malignancy
(+)
(-)
Malignancy-induced hypercalcemia
Vitamin D therapy?
✓ 25-hydroxyvitamin D level
Vitamin D intoxication
Excessive calcium ingestion?
Metabolic alkalosis?
Renal insufficiency?
Milk-alkali syndrome
See next page

HYPERCALCEMIA (*continued*)

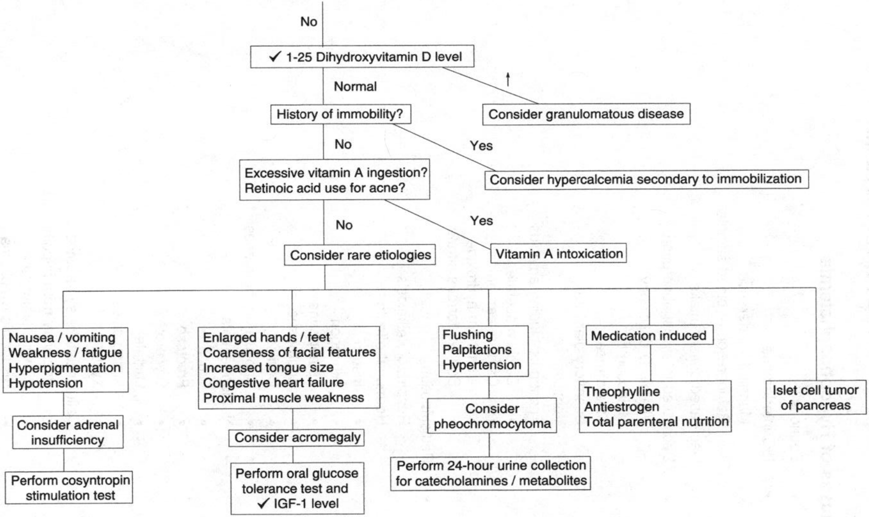
No
✓ 1-25 Dihydroxyvitamin D level
Normal
↑
Consider granulomatous disease
History of immobility?
No
Yes
Consider hypercalcemia secondary to immobilization
Excessive vitamin A ingestion?
Retinoic acid use for acne?
No
Yes
Vitamin A intoxication
Consider rare etiologies
Nausea / vomiting
Weakness / fatigue
Hyperpigmentation
Hypotension
Consider adrenal insufficiency
Perform cosyntropin stimulation test
Enlarged hands / feet
Coarseness of facial features
Increased tongue size
Congestive heart failure
Proximal muscle weakness
Consider acromegaly
Perform oral glucose tolerance test and ✓ IGF-1 level
Flushing
Palpitations
Hypertension
Consider pheochromocytoma
Perform 24-hour urine collection for catecholamines / metabolites
Medication induced
Theophylline
Antiestrogen
Total parenteral nutrition
Islet cell tumor of pancreas

HYPOPHOSPHATEMIA

Causes of Hypophosphatemia

- Spurious
- IgG interference
  - Mannitol interference
  - Refrigeration of blood sample
- Decreased dietary intake
- Decreased intestinal absorption
  - Vitamin D deficiency
  - Malabsorption
  - Steatorrhea
  - Secretory diarrhea
  - Vomiting
  - Phosphate-binding antacids
    - Calcium acetate
    - Calcium carbonate
    - Aluminum hydroxide
    - Sodium ferrous citrate
- Redistribution
  - Respiratory alkalosis
  - Hormonal effects
    - Insulin
    - Glucagon
    - Epinephrine
    - Androgens
    - Cortisol
    - Anovulatory hormones
  - Nutrient effects
    - Glucose
    - Fructose
    - Glycerol
    - Lactate
    - Amino acids
    - Xylitol
  - Cellular uptake syndromes
    - Recovery from hypothermia
    - Burkitt's lymphoma
    - Histiocytic lymphoma
    - Acute myelomonocytic leukemia
    - Acute myelogenous leukemia

- Treatment of pernicious anemia
- Treatment of iron deficiency with intravenous saccharated iron oxide
- Hungry bone syndrome

- Increased urinary excretion
  - Primary hyperparathyroidism
  - Oncogenic (associated with production of PTHrP)
  - Renal tubular defects
    - Nonacidotic and hypercalciuric proximal tubulopathy
    - Multiple myeloma
    - Renal rickets
    - Chinese crude drugs
    - Polyostotic fibrous dysplasia
    - Following renal transplantation
    - Maleic acid
    - Ifosfamide
    - Suramin
  - Aldosteronism
  - Licorice ingestion
  - Volume expansion
  - Inappropriate secretion of ADH
  - Mineralocorticoid administration
  - Corticosteroid therapy
  - Magnesium deficiency
  - Diuretics
  - Diphosphonates
  - Foscarnet
  - Bartter's syndrome
  - Gitelman's syndrome

Adapted from Seldin DW and Giebisch G, *The Kidney: Physiology and Pathophysiology*, Philadelphia, PA: Lippincott Williams and Wilkins, 2000, 1906.

HYPERPHOSPHATEMIA

Causes of Hyperphosphatemia

- Spurious
  - Thrombocytosis
  - Hyperlipidemia
  - Myeloma paraproteins
  - Stored blood
  - Mannitol
- Increased intake / Exogenous load
  - Cow's milk
  - Vitamin D intoxication
  - Phosphorus-containing laxatives / enema
  - Intravenous phosphorous administration
  - White phosphorus burns
- Increased endogenous load
  - Tumor lysis syndrome
  - Rhabdomyolysis
  - Malignant hyperthermia
  - Heat stroke
  - Lactic acidosis
  - Ketoacidosis
  - Respiratory acidosis
  - Respiratory alkalosis (chromic)
  - Bowel infarction
- Decreased excretion
  - Renal insufficiency
  - Hypoparathyroidism
  - Bisphosphonates
  - Growth hormone / acromegaly
  - Insulin-like growth factor I
  - Vitamin D intoxication
  - Vitamin A intoxication
  - Tumoral calcinosis
  - Pseudohypoparathyroidism
  - Steroid withdrawal
- Miscellaneous
  - Verapamil
  - β-blockers
  - Fluoride poisoning
  - Hemorrhagic shock
  - Sleep deprivation

Adapted from Seldin DW and Giebisch G, *The Kidney: Physiology and Pathophysiology*, Philadelphia, PA: Lippincott Williams and Wilkins, 2000, 1928.

ANION GAP

Causes of High Serum Anion Gap

- Metabolic acidosis
  - Uremia
  - Ketoacidosis (diabetic, alcoholic, starvation)
  - Lactic acidosis
  - Intoxication
    - Salicylate
    - Ethylene glycol
    - Methanol
- Dehydration or fluid loss (relatively little unmeasured anions)
- Nonketotic hyperosmolar coma
- Salts / organic acid infusion (lactate, acetate, citrate, penicillin, carbenicillin)
- Reduced unmeasured cations (magnesium, calcium, potassium)
- Alkalemia
- Laboratory error

Causes of a Low Serum Anion Gap

- Increased unmeasured cations
  - Normally present
    - Potassium
    - Calcium
    - Magnesium
  - Not normally present
    - IgG multiple myeloma
    - Polyclonal gammopathy
    - Lithium
    - Polymyxin B
- Decreased unmeasured anions
  - Hypoalbuminemia
- Sodium underestimation
  - Hyperviscosity
  - Severe hypernatremia

- Chloride overestimation
  - Hypertriglyceridemia
  - Bromide
  - Iodide
- Other reported causes
  - Renal transplantation
  - Hyponatremia

Adapted from Jurado R, del Rio C, Nasar G, et al, "Low Anion Gap," *Southern Med J*, 1998, 91(7):626.

APPROACH TO THE PATIENT WITH AN ACID-BASE DISORDER

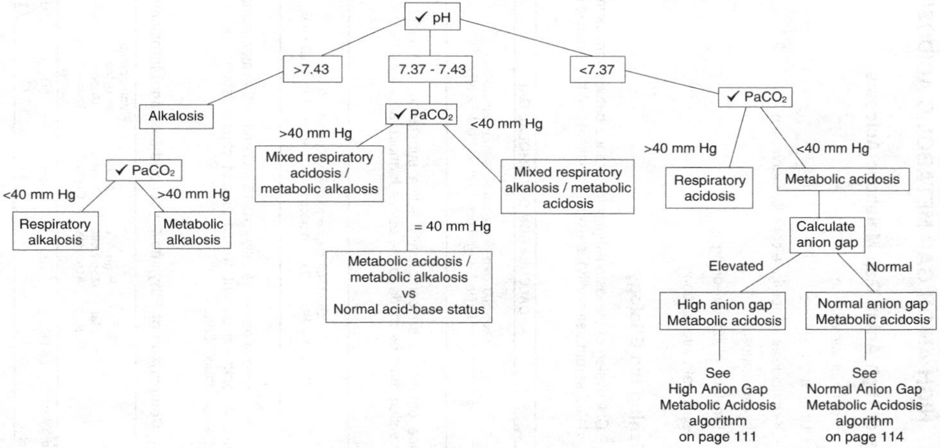
✓ pH
>7.43
7.37 - 7.43
<7.37
Alkalosis
✓ PaCO2
<40 mm Hg
>40 mm Hg
Respiratory alkalosis
Metabolic alkalosis
✓ PaCO2
>40 mm Hg
Mixed respiratory acidosis / metabolic alkalosis
<40 mm Hg
Mixed respiratory alkalosis / metabolic acidosis
= 40 mm Hg
Metabolic acidosis / metabolic alkalosis vs Normal acid-base status
✓ PaCO2
>40 mm Hg
Respiratory acidosis
<40 mm Hg
Metabolic acidosis
Calculate anion gap
Elevated
Normal
High anion gap Metabolic acidosis
Normal anion gap Metabolic acidosis
See High Anion Gap Metabolic Acidosis algorithm on page 111
See Normal Anion Gap Metabolic Acidosis algorithm on page 114

HIGH ANION GAP METABOLIC ACIDOSIS

Causes of High Anion Gap Metabolic Acidosis

- Methanol intoxication
- Uremia
- Ketoacidosis (diabetic, alcoholic, starvation)
- Lactic acidosis
- Ethylene glycol poisoning
- Salicylate intoxication

Establishing the Etiology

- Calculation of the osmolal gap (difference between measured and calculated serum osmolality) is useful in patients with metabolic acidosis

CALCULATION OF OSMOLAL GAP
Osmolal gap = measured serum osmolality - $[2(Na^+) + (glucose / 18) + (BUN / 2.8)]$

Since ethanol is an osmotically active substance, if ethanol is present, a correction must be made to the above formula, as shown below:

Osmolal gap = measured osmolality - $[2(Na^+) + BUN / 2.8 + glucose / 18 + ethanol (mg/dL) / 4.6]$

A normal osmolal gap is usually <10-15 mOsm/kg. Elevated osmolal gap in the metabolic acidosis patient should prompt consideration of ethylene glycol or methanol intoxication.

Comparison of Ethylene Glycol and Methanol Intoxication

	↑ Osmolal Gap	High AG Metabolic Acidosis	Urine Oxalate Crystals	Fluorescence of Urine Under Wood's Lamp	ARF	Optic Nerve Swelling
Ethylene glycol	(+)	(+)	(+)	(+)	(+)	(-)
Methanol	(+)	(+)	(-)	(-)	(-)	(+)

- If the osmolal gap is normal, other causes of high anion gap metabolic acidosis should be considered such as uremia, ketoacidosis, salicylate intoxication, and lactic acidosis.
- Uremia is usually apparent but the clinician should realize that other causes of high anion gap metabolic acidosis may be present in the uremic patient.
- The three types of ketoacidosis include diabetic, alcoholic, and starvation. To establish the diagnosis of ketoacidosis, it is necessary to demonstrate the presence of ketones in the blood or urine. Criteria for the diagnosis of diabetic ketoacidosis is listed in the following box.

CRITERIA FOR DIAGNOSIS OF DKA	
GLUCOSE >250 mg/dL	pH <7.3
HCO_3^- <15 mEq/L	KETONEMIA / KETONURIA
HIGH ANION GAP METABOLIC ACIDOSIS	

- Patients with salicylate intoxication often have complex acid-base abnormalities. A pure metabolic acidosis is uncommon and many patients have a combined respiratory alkalosis and metabolic acidosis.
- Causes of lactic acidosis are listed below.

  Type A

  - Seizures
  - Severe exercise
  - Shock / hypotension
    - Cardiogenic
    - Hypovolemic
    - Sepsis
    - Anaphylaxis
    - Massive pulmonary embolism
  - Severe hypoxemia
    - Carbon monoxide poisoning
    - Severe anemia
    - Methemoglobinemia
    - Acute respiratory failure

  Type B

  - Drugs / toxins
    - Metformin

- Acetaminophen
- Niacin
- Lactulose
- Theophylline
- Cocaine
- Papaverine
- Sorbitol
- Ethanol
- Salicylates
- Cyanide
- Methanol
- Isoniazid
- Nitroprusside
- Streptozotocin
- Ethylene glycol
- Nalidixic acid
- Others

– Infection
  – Malaria
  – Cholera
– Malignancy
  – Leukemia
  – Lymphoma
  – Solid cancers
– Inherited enzyme defects
– Renal failure
– Diabetes mellitus
– Liver failure
– Sepsis
– D-lactic acidosis

HIGH ANION GAP METABOLIC ACIDOSIS

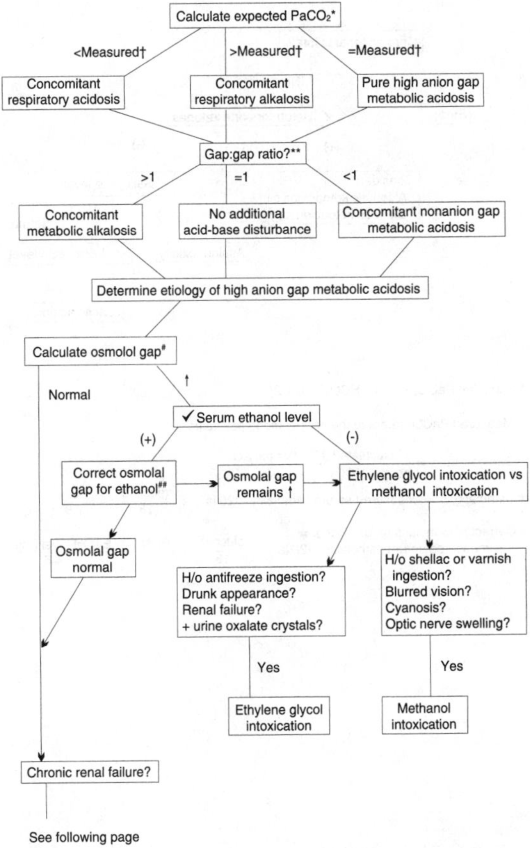
Calculate expected PaCO₂*
<Measured†
>Measured†
=Measured†
Concomitant respiratory acidosis
Concomitant respiratory alkalosis
Pure high anion gap metabolic acidosis
Gap:gap ratio?**
>1
=1
<1
Concomitant metabolic alkalosis
No additional acid-base disturbance
Concomitant nonanion gap metabolic acidosis
Determine etiology of high anion gap metabolic acidosis
Calculate osmolol gap#
Normal
↑
✓ Serum ethanol level
(+)
(-)
Correct osmolal gap for ethanol##
Osmolal gap remains ↑
Ethylene glycol intoxication vs methanol intoxication
Osmolal gap normal
H/o antifreeze ingestion?
Drunk appearance?
Renal failure?
+ urine oxalate crystals?
H/o shellac or varnish ingestion?
Blurred vision?
Cyanosis?
Optic nerve swelling?
Yes
Yes
Ethylene glycol intoxication
Methanol intoxication
Chronic renal failure?
See following page

HIGH ANION GAP METABOLIC ACIDOSIS (*continued*)

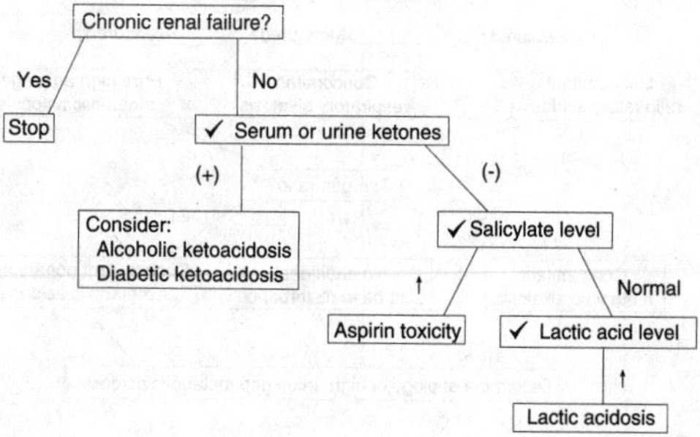
Chronic renal failure?
Yes
No
Stop
✓ Serum or urine ketones
(+)
(-)
Consider:
Alcoholic ketoacidosis
Diabetic ketoacidosis
✓ Salicylate level
↑
Normal
Aspirin toxicity
✓ Lactic acid level
↑
Lactic acidosis

* Expected $PaCO_2 = [1.5 \times HCO_3^- + 8 \pm 2]$

† Measured $PaCO_2$ refers to the arterial blood gas value

** Gap:gap ratio $= \dfrac{\text{calculated AG - normal AG}}{\text{normal } HCO_3^- \text{ - measured } HCO_3^-}$

Osmolal gap = measured serum osmolality - $[2(Na^+) + \dfrac{\text{glucose}}{18} + \dfrac{\text{BUN}}{2.8}]$

Corrected osmolal gap for alcohol =
measured serum osmolality - $[2(Na^+) + \dfrac{\text{glucose}}{18} + \dfrac{\text{BUN}}{2.8} + \dfrac{\text{ETOH level (mg/dL)}}{4.6}]$

NORMAL ANION GAP METABOLIC ACIDOSIS

Causes of Normal Anion Gap Metabolic Acidosis

- Renal tubular acidosis
  - Associated with hypokalemia
    - Distal renal tubular acidosis (type I)
    - Proximal renal tubular acidosis (type II)
  - Associated with hyperkalemia
    - Type IV renal tubular acidosis
    - Medication-induced
      - Amiloride
      - Triamterene
      - Spironolactone
      - Trimethoprim
      - Pentamidine
      - ACE inhibitor
      - Angiotensin II receptor blocker
      - NSAIDs
      - Cyclosporine
  - Associated with normokalemia (early renal failure)
- Gastrointestinal loss of alkali
  - Diarrhea
  - Pancreatic fistula
  - Biliary fistula
  - Enteric fistula
  - Pancreatic transplantation with drainage into urinary bladder
  - Ureterosigmoidostomy
  - Jejunal loop
  - Medications
    - Calcium chloride
    - Magnesium sulfate
    - Cholestyramine
- Miscellaneous
  - Recovery from ketoacidosis
  - Posthypocapnia
  - Expansion acidosis
  - Cation exchange resins

NORMAL ANION GAP METABOLIC ACIDOSIS

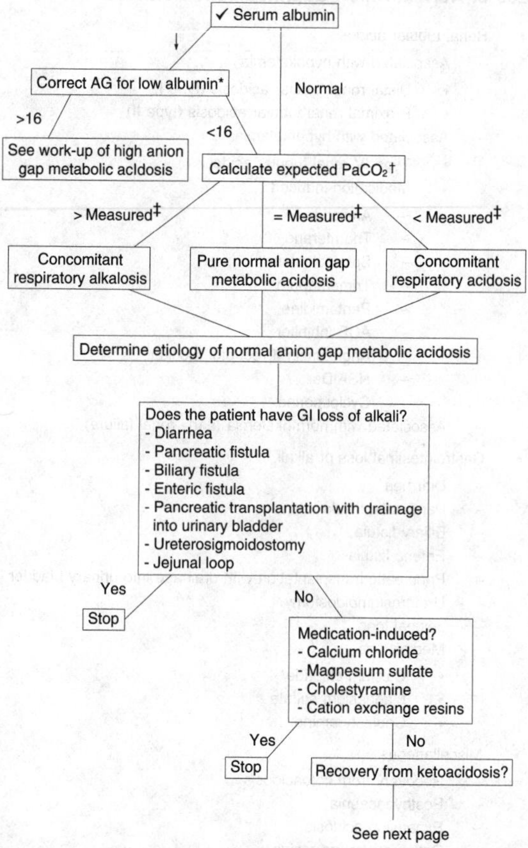
✓ Serum albumin
Correct AG for low albumin*
Normal
>16
<16
See work-up of high anion gap metabolic acidosis
Calculate expected PaCO2†
> Measured‡
= Measured‡
< Measured‡
Concomitant respiratory alkalosis
Pure normal anion gap metabolic acidosis
Concomitant respiratory acidosis
Determine etiology of normal anion gap metabolic acidosis
Does the patient have GI loss of alkali?
- Diarrhea
- Pancreatic fistula
- Biliary fistula
- Enteric fistula
- Pancreatic transplantation with drainage into urinary bladder
- Ureterosigmoidostomy
- Jejunal loop
Yes
Stop
No
Medication-induced?
- Calcium chloride
- Magnesium sulfate
- Cholestyramine
- Cation exchange resins
Yes
Stop
No
Recovery from ketoacidosis?
See next page

NORMAL ANION GAP METABOLIC ACIDOSIS *(continued)*

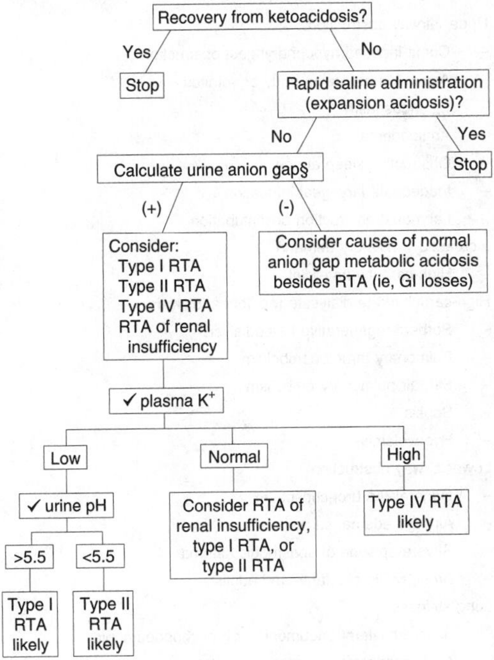
Recovery from ketoacidosis?
Yes
Stop
No
Rapid saline administration (expansion acidosis)?
No
Yes
Stop
Calculate urine anion gap§
(+)
(-)
Consider: Type I RTA Type II RTA Type IV RTA RTA of renal insufficiency
Consider causes of normal anion gap metabolic acidosis besides RTA (ie, GI losses)
✓ plasma K+
Low
Normal
High
✓ urine pH
Consider RTA of renal insufficiency, type I RTA, or type II RTA
Type IV RTA likely
>5.5
<5.5
Type I RTA likely
Type II RTA likely

* Corrected AG = $AG_{measured}$ + 2.5 (4-albumin)

† Expected $PaCO_2 = [(1.5 \times HCO_3^-) + 8 \pm 2]$

‡ Measured $PaCO_2$ refers to the arterial blood gas value

§ Urine AG = $U_{Na^+} + U_{K^+} - U_{Cl^-}$

RESPIRATORY ACIDOSIS

Causes of Acute Respiratory Acidosis

- Upper airway obstruction
  - Coma-induced hypopharyngeal obstruction
  - Aspiration of foreign body or vomitus
  - Laryngospasm
  - Angioedema
  - Obstructive sleep apnea
  - Inadequate laryngeal intubation
  - Laryngeal obstruction postintubation
- Increased ventilatory demand
  - High-carbohydrate diet
- High-carbohydrate dialysate (peritoneal dialysis)
  - Sorbent-regenerative hemodialysis
  - Pulmonary thromboembolism
  - Fat, air pulmonary embolism
  - Sepsis
  - Hypovolemia
- Lower airway obstruction
  - Generalized bronchospasm
  - Airways edema, secretions
  - Severe episode of spasmodic asthma
  - Bronchiolitis of infants and adults
- Lung stiffness
  - Severe bilateral pneumonia or bronchopneumonia
  - Acute respiratory distress syndrome
  - Severe pulmonary edema
  - Atelectasis
- Chest wall stiffness
  - Rib fractures with flail chest
  - Pneumothorax
  - Hemothorax
  - Abdominal distention

  - Ascites
  - Peritoneal dialysis
- Muscle dysfunction
  - Fatigue
  - Hyperkalemia
  - Hypokalemia
  - Hypoperfusion state
  - Hypoxemia
  - Malnutrition
- Depressed central drive
  - General anesthesia
  - Sedative overdose
  - Head trauma
  - CVA
  - Central sleep apnea
  - Cerebral edema
  - Brain tumor
  - Encephalitis
  - Brainstem lesion
- Abnormal neuromuscular transmission
  - High spinal cord injury
  - Guillan-Barré syndrome
  - Status epilepticus
  - Botulism
  - Tetanus
  - Crisis in myasthenia gravis
- Hypokalemic myopathy
  - Familial periodic paralysis
  - Drugs / toxic agents (curare, succinylcholine, aminoglycosides, organophosphorus)

Adapted from Johnson R and Feehally J, *Comprehensive Clinical Nephrology*, Harcourt Publishers Ltd, 2000, 3.14.2

Causes of Chronic Respiratory Acidosis

- Upper airway obstruction
  - Tonsillar and peritonsillar hypertrophy
  - Paralysis of the vocal cords
  - Tumor of the cords or larynx
  - Airway stenosis postprolonged intubation
  - Thymoma
  - Aortic aneurysm
- Lower airway obstruction
  - Airway scarring
  - Chronic obstructive lung disease
    - Bronchitis
    - Bronchiolitis
    - Bronchiectasis
    - Emphysema
- Lung stiffness
  - Severe chronic pneumonitis
  - Diffuse infiltrative disease (eg, alveolar proteinosis)
  - Interstitial fibrosis
- Chest wall stiffness
  - Kyphoscoliosis
  - Spinal arthritis
  - Obesity
  - Fibrothorax
  - Hydrothorax
  - Chest wall tumors
- Muscle dysfunction (eg, polymyositis)
- Depressed central drive
  - Sedative overdose
  - Methadone / heroin addiction
  - Sleep disordered breathing
  - Brain tumor
  - Bulbar poliomyelitis
  - Hypothyroidism

- Abnormal neuromuscular transmission
  - Poliomyelitis
  - Multiple sclerosis
  - Muscular dystrophy
  - Amyotrophic lateral sclerosis
  - Diaphragmatic paralysis
  - Myopathic disease (polymyositis)

Adapted from Johnson R and Feehally J, *Comprehensive Clinical Nephrology*, Harcourt Publishers Ltd, 2000, 3.14.2.

RESPIRATORY ALKALOSIS

Causes of Respiratory Alkalosis

- CNS event
  - CVA
  - Infection (meningitis, encephalitis)
  - Tumor
  - Trauma
  - Fever
  - Psychosis
  - Pain
  - Anxiety
  - Hyperventilation syndrome
- Drug use
  - Salicylates
  - Progesterone
  - Nicotine
  - Methylxanthines
  - Catecholamines
- Lung disease
- Interstitial lung disease
  - Pulmonary edema (cardiogenic or noncardiogenic)
  - Pneumonia
  - Pulmonary embolism
  - Asthma
  - Pneumothorax
  - Aspiration
  - Flail chest
- Miscellaneous
  - Pregnancy
  - Sepsis
  - Liver cirrhosis or failure
  - Hemodialysis with acetate dialysis
  - Heat exposure
  - Severe anemia
  - Hyperthyroidism
  - High altitude
  - Right to left shunt
  - Aspiration
  - Laryngospasm

METABOLIC ALKALOSIS

Causes of Metabolic Alkalosis

- Exogenous alkali
  - Antacids
  - Citrate
- Intravenous lactate
  - Massive blood transfusion
  - Plasmapheresis
- Nonabsorbable antacids with exchange resin
- Milk-alkali syndrome
- Refeeding syndrome
- Hypercalcemia
- Chloride-responsive metabolic alkalosis
  - Vomiting or other gastric loss
  - Chloride-losing diarrhea
  - Villous adenoma
  - Diuretic therapy (remote)
  - Poorly reabsorbable anions
  - Posthypercapnia
- Chloride-unresponsive metabolic alkalosis
  - Primary hyperaldosteronism
  - Renal artery stenosis
  - Renin-secreting tumor
  - Malignant hypertension
  - Cushing's syndrome
  - Exogenous mineralocorticoids
  - Adrenal enzyme deficiencies
  - Liddle's syndrome
  - Bartter's syndrome
  - Gitelman's syndrome
  - Magnesium deficiency
  - Potassium deficiency
  - Diuretic therapy

METABOLIC ALKALOSIS

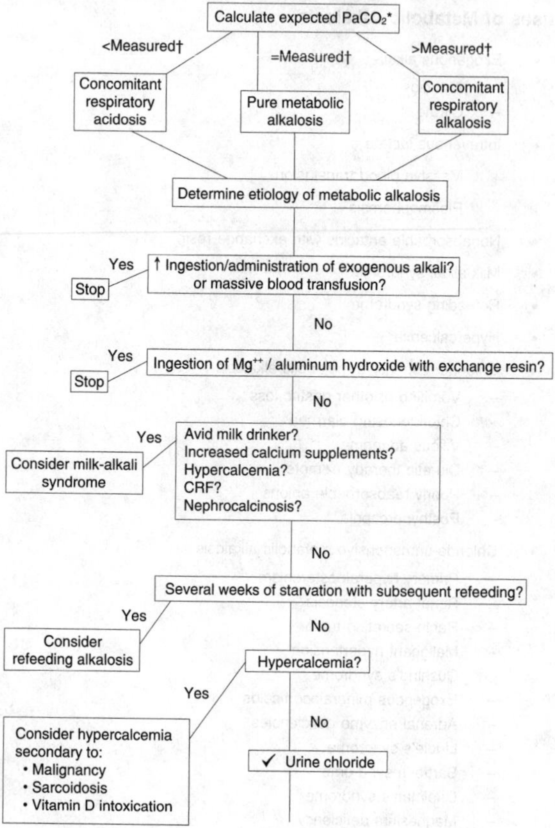
Calculate expected PaCO2*
<Measured†
=Measured†
>Measured†
Concomitant respiratory acidosis
Pure metabolic alkalosis
Concomitant respiratory alkalosis
Determine etiology of metabolic alkalosis
Yes
Stop
↑ Ingestion/administration of exogenous alkali? or massive blood transfusion?
No
Yes
Stop
Ingestion of Mg++ / aluminum hydroxide with exchange resin?
No
Yes
Consider milk-alkali syndrome
Avid milk drinker?
Increased calcium supplements?
Hypercalcemia?
CRF?
Nephrocalcinosis?
No
Several weeks of starvation with subsequent refeeding?
Yes
Consider refeeding alkalosis
No
Hypercalcemia?
Yes
Consider hypercalcemia secondary to:
• Malignancy
• Sarcoidosis
• Vitamin D intoxication
No
✓ Urine chloride

See following page

METABOLIC ALKALOSIS *(continued)*

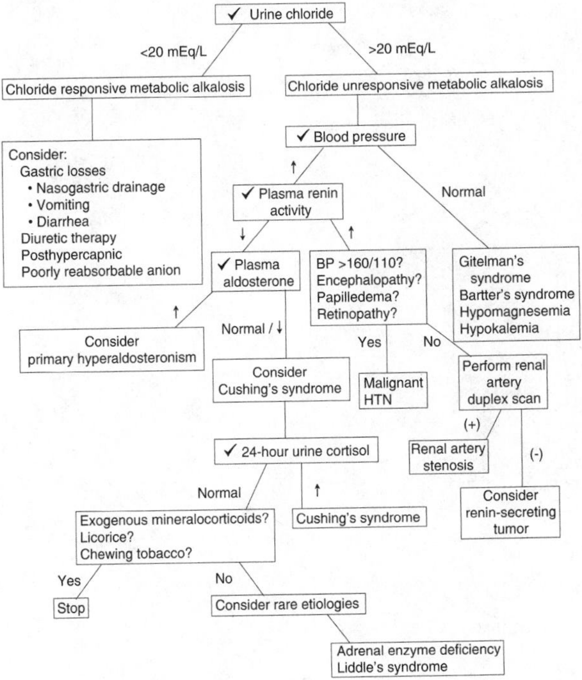
✓ Urine chloride
<20 mEq/L
>20 mEq/L
Chloride responsive metabolic alkalosis
Chloride unresponsive metabolic alkalosis
Consider:
Gastric losses
• Nasogastric drainage
• Vomiting
• Diarrhea
Diuretic therapy
Posthypercapnic
Poorly reabsorbable anion
✓ Blood pressure
↑
Normal
✓ Plasma renin activity
↓
↑
✓ Plasma aldosterone
BP >160/110?
Encephalopathy?
Papilledema?
Retinopathy?
Gitelman's syndrome
Bartter's syndrome
Hypomagnesemia
Hypokalemia
↑
Consider primary hyperaldosteronism
Normal / ↓
Yes
No
Consider Cushing's syndrome
Malignant HTN
Perform renal artery duplex scan
(+)
Renal artery stenosis
(-)
✓ 24-hour urine cortisol
Normal
↑
Consider renin-secreting tumor
Exogenous mineralocorticoids?
Licorice?
Chewing tobacco?
Cushing's syndrome
Yes
No
Stop
Consider rare etiologies
Adrenal enzyme deficiency
Liddle's syndrome

* Expected $PaCO_2 = HCO_3^- + 15$

† Measured $PaCO_2$ refers to the arterial blood gas value

ENDOCRINE

ADRENAL INSUFFICIENCY

Diagnosis of Adrenal Insufficiency

- The two tests that are often obtained to establish the diagnosis of adrenal insufficiency are the AM serum cortisol level and the short ACTH stimulation test (cosyntropin). These tests are discussed below.

AM Serum Cortisol

- The evaluation of the patient suspected of having adrenal insufficiency often begins with measurement of the AM serum cortisol level.
- Serum cortisol levels are normally at their highest in the early morning (4-8 AM). There is no point in measuring serum cortisol levels in the late afternoon or evening because levels are normally low at this time.
- Therefore, in the patient suspected of having adrenal insufficiency, a low AM serum cortisol level (<3 μg/dL) provides strong support for the diagnosis. A level <10 μg/dL is strongly suggestive of adrenal insufficiency (sensitivity 62%, specificity 77%).

Short ACTH Stimulation Test (Cosyntropin Stimulation Test)

- Many clinicians bypass measurement of the AM serum cortisol level and proceed directly to the cosyntropin stimulation test when adrenal insufficiency is suspected.
- Even in patients who have an AM serum cortisol level measured, the cosyntropin stimulation test is often performed either because the AM serum cortisol level was not consistent with adrenal insufficiency or if a low level was obtained, confirmation of the diagnosis is required.
- Most experts recommend that this test be performed in almost all patients suspected of having adrenal insufficiency.
- In the standard test, 250 μg of ACTH is given (I.M./I.V.) and the serum cortisol level is measured after 30 or 60 minutes.
- A normal response is defined as a peak of 18-20 μg/dL or more.
- A subnormal response establishes the diagnosis of adrenal insufficiency.
- A normal response excludes primary adrenal insufficiency and most cases of secondary adrenal insufficiency. If secondary adrenal insufficiency is of recent onset, however, test results may be normal. In these cases, the

insulin-induced hypoglycemia or metapyrone test is needed to establish the diagnosis.

- In patients with adrenal crisis, treatment should not be delayed in order to perform the cosyntropin stimulation test. The stimulation test can be performed after starting therapy as long as it is done within the first few days of treatment and the patient is not receiving hydrocortisone. Hydrocortisone can interfere with the serum cortisol measurement.

Differentiating Primary From Secondary / Tertiary Adrenal Insufficiency

- Once the diagnosis of adrenal insufficiency has been established, the clinician should perform testing to differentiate primary from secondary/ tertiary adrenal insufficiency.
- Quite often, this evaluation begins with measurement of the basal plasma ACTH.
- In primary adrenal insufficiency, the 8 AM plasma ACTH is high. In secondary or tertiary adrenal insufficiency, the plasma ACTH level is low or low normal.
- Because glucocorticoid therapy will suppress ACTH secretion, blood samples for ACTH measurement must be obtained before starting therapy. If this is not possible, the ACTH level should not be obtained until at least 24 hours have passed since the last dose of a short-acting glucocorticoid such as hydrocortisone. An even longer interval of time should pass before testing occurs in the patient receiving a longer-acting agent such as dexamethasone.

ADRENAL INSUFFICIENCY

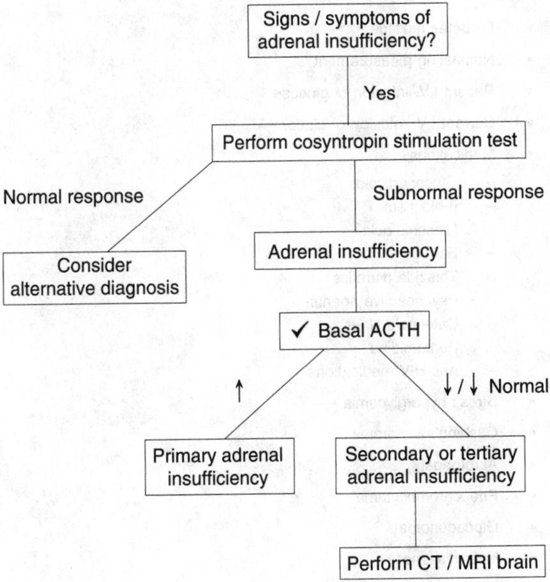
Signs / symptoms of adrenal insufficiency?
Yes
Perform cosyntropin stimulation test
Normal response
Subnormal response
Consider alternative diagnosis
Adrenal insufficiency
✓ Basal ACTH
↑
↓ / ↓ Normal
Primary adrenal insufficiency
Secondary or tertiary adrenal insufficiency
Perform CT / MRI brain

HYPERGLYCEMIA

Causes of Hyperglycemia

- Diabetes mellitus
- Nonfasting measurement
- Recent I.V. infusion of glucose
- Current I.V. infusion of glucose
- Medications
  - Glucocorticoids
  - β-blockers
  - Nicotinic acid
  - Estrogens
  - Thiazide diuretics
  - Psychoactive agents
  - Catecholamines
  - Pentamidine
  - Anti-HIV medications
- Stress hyperglycemia
- Cushing's syndrome
- Acromegaly
- Pheochromocytoma
- Glucagonoma
- Liver disease
- Pancreatitis
- Pancreatectomy
- Cystic fibrosis
- Hemochromatosis

Establishing the Diagnosis of Diabetes Mellitus

CRITERIA FOR THE DIAGNOSIS OF DIABETES MELLITUS
1) Symptoms of diabetes plus casual plasma glucose ≥200 mg/dL* (11.1 mmol/L)
or
2) Fasting plasma glucose ≥126 mg/dL† (7 mmol/L)
or
3) Two-hour plasma glucose ≥200 mg/dL (11.1 mmol/L) during an observed glucose tolerance test (OGTT)‡

*Casual is defined as any time of the day without regard to time since a last meal. The classic symptoms of diabetes include polyuria, polydipsia, and unexplained weight loss.

†Fasting is defined as no caloric intake for at least 8 hours.

‡The test should be performed as described by WHO, using a glucose load containing the equivalent of 75 g of anhydrous glucose dissolved in water.

Obtained with permission from the Report of the Expert Committee on the Diagnosis and Classification of Diabetes Mellitus, *Diabetes Care*, 1997, 20(7):1183-97.

Severe Hyperglycemia

- The presence of severe hyperglycemia should always prompt consideration of diabetic ketoacidosis and nonketotic hyperosmolar syndrome.

CHARACTERISTIC CLINICAL FINDINGS IN DIABETIC KETOACIDOSIS AND NONKETOTIC HYPEROSMOLAR SYNDROME

Finding	Diabetic Ketoacidosis	Nonketotic Hyperosmolar Syndrome
Age	Young (less commonly elderly)	Middle-aged to elderly
Type of diabetes	Type 1 (less often type 2)	Type 2
Onset	Acute or subacute	Insidious
Abdominal pain	Yes	No
Kussmaul's respiration	Yes	No
Acetone in breath	Yes	No
Temperature	Normothermic or hypothermic	Normothermic or hyperthermic
Volume depletion	Moderate	Severe
Blood pressure	Normotensive	Orthostatic hypotension
Change in mental status	Moderate	Severe (coma or seizures)

Adapted from Jabbour SA and Miller JL, "Uncontrolled Diabetes Mellitus," *Clin Lab Med*, 2001, 21(1):102.

LABORATORY TEST FINDINGS IN DIABETIC KETOACIDOSIS AND NONKETOTIC HYPEROSMOLAR SYNDROME

Finding	Diabetic Ketoacidosis	Nonketotic Hyperosmolar Syndrome
Plasma glucose	>250 mg/dL	>600 mg/dL
Plasma osmolality	<330 mOsm/kg	>330 mOsm/kg
Ketones		
urine	>+3	- or small amounts
blood	+ at >1:2 dilution	- or small amounts
Serum bicarbonate	<15 mEq/L	>20 mEq/L
pH	<7.30	>7.30
BUN	<25 mg/dL	>30 mg/dL

Glycosylated Hemoglobin

- Glycosylated hemoglobin (HB AIc) is a measure of overall blood glucose control over a period of 60-120 days.
- Measurement is recommended in every patient with diabetes mellitus at the time of diagnosis.
- In diabetes mellitus, clinicians often measure levels every 3-6 months.
- The American Diabetes Association has recommended that clinicians strive for a level <7% in diabetes mellitus patients.
- Therapy should be reevaluated if levels are consistently >8%.

HYPOGLYCEMIA

Causes of Hypoglycemia

- **Fasting**
  - Pancreatic disease
    - Insulinoma
  - Liver disease
    - Cirrhosis
    - Hepatitis
    - Carcinomatosis
    - Ascending cholangitis
    - Circulatory failure
  - Renal disease
  - CNS disease
    - Hypothalamic disease
    - Brainstem disease
  - Pituitary disease
    - Hypopituitarism
  - Adrenal disease
    - Adrenal insufficiency
    - Congenital adrenal hyperplasia
  - Nonpancreatic malignancy
  - Medications
  - Sepsis
  - Miscellaneous
    - Prolonged strenuous exercise
  - Autoimmune hypoglycemia
    - Pregnancy
    - Lactation
    - Diarrheal states
    - Chronic starvation
- **Reactive**
  - Alimentary hypoglycemia
  - Idiopathic postprandial (functional)

HYPOGLYCEMIA

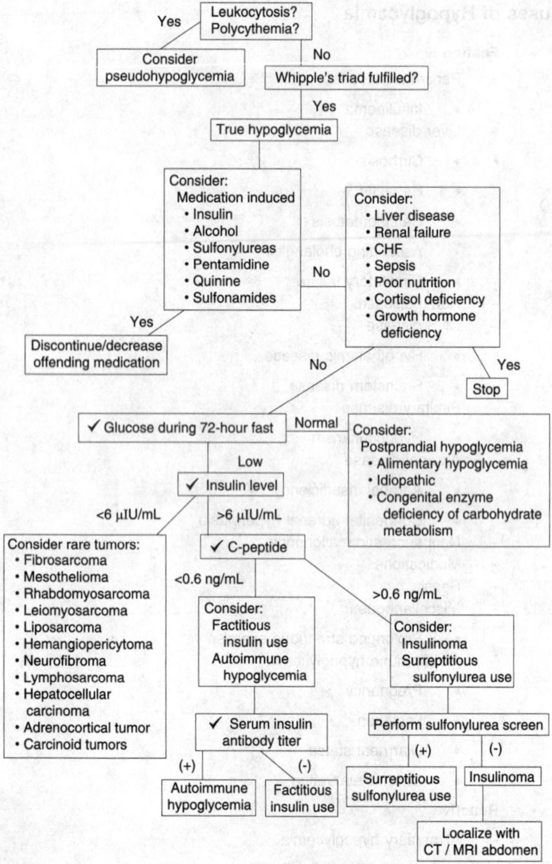
Leukocytosis? Polycythemia?
Yes
Consider pseudohypoglycemia
No
Whipple's triad fulfilled?
Yes
True hypoglycemia
Consider:
Medication induced
• Insulin
• Alcohol
• Sulfonylureas
• Pentamidine
• Quinine
• Sulfonamides
No
Consider:
• Liver disease
• Renal failure
• CHF
• Sepsis
• Poor nutrition
• Cortisol deficiency
• Growth hormone deficiency
Yes
Discontinue/decrease offending medication
No
Yes
Stop
✓ Glucose during 72-hour fast
Normal
Consider:
Postprandial hypoglycemia
• Alimentary hypoglycemia
• Idiopathic
• Congenital enzyme deficiency of carbohydrate metabolism
Low
✓ Insulin level
<6 μIU/mL
>6 μIU/mL
Consider rare tumors:
• Fibrosarcoma
• Mesothelioma
• Rhabdomyosarcoma
• Leiomyosarcoma
• Liposarcoma
• Hemangiopericytoma
• Neurofibroma
• Lymphosarcoma
• Hepatocellular carcinoma
• Adrenocortical tumor
• Carcinoid tumors
✓ C-peptide
<0.6 ng/mL
>0.6 ng/mL
Consider:
Factitious insulin use
Autoimmune hypoglycemia
Consider:
Insulinoma
Surreptitious sulfonylurea use
✓ Serum insulin antibody titer
(+)
(-)
Autoimmune hypoglycemia
Factitious insulin use
Perform sulfonylurea screen
(+)
(-)
Surreptitious sulfonylurea use
Insulinoma
Localize with CT / MRI abdomen

APPROACH TO THE PATIENT WITH ELEVATED TSH

Causes of Elevated TSH

- Primary hypothyroidism
- Subclinical hypothyroidism
- Recovery phase of nonthyroidal illness
- Inadequate thyroid hormone replacement
- Malabsorption of oral thyroid hormone
- Drug inhibition of thyroid hormone secretion
- Intermittent compliance with thyroid hormone therapy
- Adrenal insufficiency
- TSH-producing pituitary adenoma
- Thyroid hormone resistance

Causes of Elevated TSH and Decreased Free T_4 Levels

- Primary hypothyroidism
- Inadequate thyroid hormone replacement
- Drug inhibition of thyroid hormone secretion
- Malabsorption of oral thyroid hormone
- Recovery from nonthyroidal illness

Causes of Elevated TSH and Normal Free T_4 Levels

- Subclinical hypothyroidism
- Recovery phase of nonthyroidal illness
- Poor compliance with oral thyroid hormone replacement
- Adrenal insufficiency

Causes of Elevated TSH and Increased Free T_4 Levels

- TSH-producing pituitary adenoma
- Thyroid hormone resistance

APPROACH TO ↑ TSH LEVEL

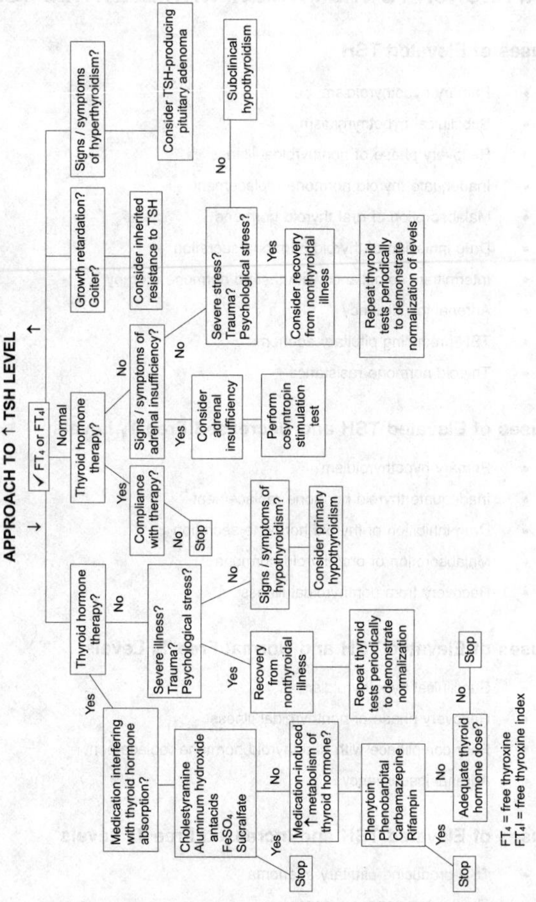
✓ FT4 or FT4I
↓
Normal
↑
Thyroid hormone therapy?
Yes
No
Medication interfering with thyroid hormone absorption?
Cholestyramine
Aluminum hydroxide antacids
FeSO4
Sucralfate
Yes
Stop
No
Medication-induced ↑ metabolism of thyroid hormone?
Phenytoin
Phenobarbital
Carbamazepine
Rifampin
Yes
Stop
No
Adequate thyroid hormone dose?
No
Stop
Severe illness?
Trauma?
Psychological stress?
Yes
Recovery from nonthyroidal illness
Repeat thyroid tests periodically to demonstrate normalization
No
Signs / symptoms of hypothyroidism?
Consider primary hypothyroidism
Thyroid hormone therapy?
Yes
Compliance with therapy?
No
Stop
No
Signs / symptoms of adrenal insufficiency?
Yes
Consider adrenal insufficiency
Perform cosyntropin stimulation test
No
Severe stress?
Trauma?
Psychological stress?
Yes
Consider recovery from nonthyroidal illness
Repeat thyroid tests periodically to demonstrate normalization of levels
No
Subclinical hypothyroidism
Growth retardation?
Goiter?
Consider inherited resistance to TSH
Signs / symptoms of hyperthyroidism?
Consider TSH-producing pituitary adenoma

FT_4 = free thyroxine
FT_4I = free thyroxine index

APPROACH TO THE PATIENT WITH DECREASED TSH

Causes of Decreased TSH

- Hyperthyroidism
- Subclinical hyperthyroidism
- Excessive thyroid hormone replacement
- Acute psychiatric illness
- Nonthyroidal illness
- Drug inhibition of TSH release
- Pituitary failure
- T_3 thyrotoxicosis
- Pregnancy

Causes of Decreased TSH and Increased Free T_4 Levels

- Excessive oral thyroid hormone replacement
- Acute psychiatric illness
- Hyperthyroidism

Causes of Decreased TSH and Normal Free T_4 Levels

- Pregnancy
- Subclinical hyperthyroidism
- T_3 thyrotoxicosis
- Excessive oral thyroid hormone replacement
- Acute psychiatric illness
- Drug inhibition of TSH release (corticosteroid, dopamine)

Causes of Decreased TSH and Decreased Free T_4 Levels

- Nonthyroidal illness
- Pituitary failure

APPROACH TO ↓ TSH

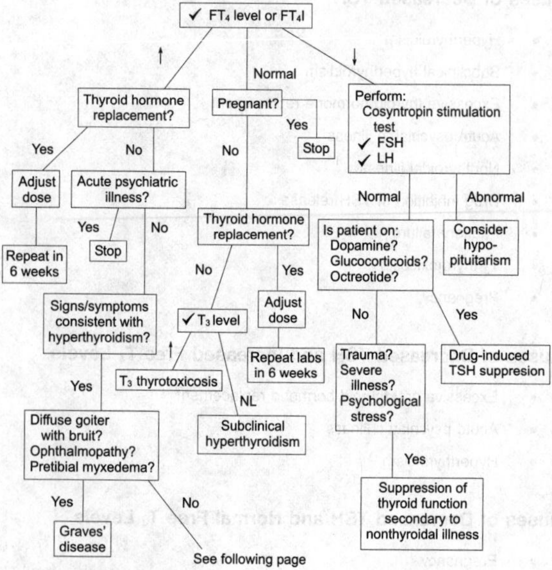
✓ FT₄ level or FT₄I
↑
Normal
↓
Thyroid hormone replacement?
Pregnant?
Yes
Stop
Perform: Cosyntropin stimulation test ✓ FSH ✓ LH
Yes
No
No
Adjust dose
Acute psychiatric illness?
Normal
Abnormal
Yes
No
Thyroid hormone replacement?
Is patient on: Dopamine? Glucocorticoids? Octreotide?
Consider hypo-pituitarism
Repeat in 6 weeks
Stop
No
Yes
Signs/symptoms consistent with hyperthyroidism?
✓ T₃ level
Adjust dose
No
Yes
↑
Repeat labs in 6 weeks
Trauma? Severe illness? Psychological stress?
Drug-induced TSH suppresion
T₃ thyrotoxicosis
Yes
NL
Diffuse goiter with bruit? Ophthalmopathy? Pretibial myxedema?
Subclinical hyperthyroidism
Yes
Suppression of thyroid function secondary to nonthyroidal illness
Yes
No
Graves' disease
See following page

FT₄ = free thyroxine
FT₄I = free thyroxine index

APPROACH TO ↓ TSH (*continued*)

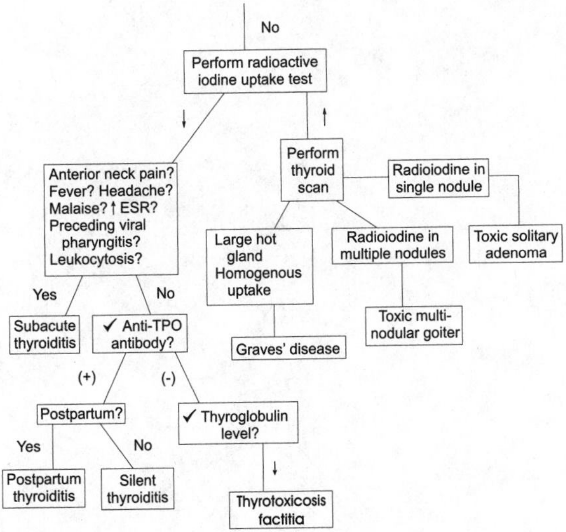
No
Perform radioactive iodine uptake test
↓
↑
Anterior neck pain? Fever? Headache? Malaise? ↑ ESR? Preceding viral pharyngitis? Leukocytosis?
Yes
No
Subacute thyroiditis
✓ Anti-TPO antibody?
(+)
(-)
Postpartum?
Yes
No
Postpartum thyroiditis
Silent thyroiditis
✓ Thyroglobulin level?
↓
Thyrotoxicosis factitia
Perform thyroid scan
Radioiodine in single nodule
Toxic solitary adenoma
Large hot gland Homogenous uptake
Graves' disease
Radioiodine in multiple nodules
Toxic multi-nodular goiter

PULMONARY

PLEURAL FLUID ANALYSIS

Analysis of the pleural fluid begins with efforts to differentiate between transudative and exudative pleural effusion. To make this distinction, the following tests need to be obtained:

- Serum protein level
- Pleural fluid protein level
- Serum LDH
- Pleural fluid LDH

These tests form the basis of Light's criteria which are used to separate transudative from exudative pleural effusions.

Light's Criteria for Exudative Pleural Effusion*

- Pleural fluid to serum protein ratio >0.5
- Pleural fluid to serum LDH ratio >0.6
- Pleural fluid LDH >2/3 upper limit of normal serum LDH

*Only one of the above criteria needs to be met for the effusion to be classified as exudative.

Tests to Order on Pleural Fluid

In patients who are found to have an exudative pleural effusion, the following tests of the pleural fluid are routinely indicated:

- Glucose
- Amylase
- Differential cell count
- Microbiologic studies
- Cytologic studies

Other tests such as pH, complement levels, lipid analysis, and rheumatoid factor should not be obtained in every patient but should be individualized depending upon the patient's clinical presentation.

Gross Appearance

- *Bloody*: Consider trauma, malignancy, pulmonary infarct, postcardiac injury syndrome, tuberculosis, asbestos-related

- *Milky*: Consider chylothorax, chyliform (pseudochylothorax)
- *Anchovy paste consistency*: Amebic infection
- *Color of enteral feed*: Misplacement of feeding tube in pleural space
- *Putrid odor*: Empyema from anaerobic infection
- *Ammonia-like odor*: Urinothorax

White Blood Cell Count and Differential

- *Neutrophilia*: Consider pneumonia, pulmonary embolism, subphrenic abscess, pancreatitis, early tuberculosis
- *Eosinophilia*: Consider air or blood in pleural space, parasitic infection (paragonimiasis, hyatid disease, amebiasis, ascariasis), medication reaction (dantrolene, nitrofurantoin, bromocriptine), Churg-Strauss syndrome, asbestos-related effusion
- *Lymphocytosis*: Consider malignancy, tuberculosis

Glucose

Causes of low pleural fluid glucose level (<60 mg/dL) include:

- Malignancy
- Hemothorax
- Tuberculosis
- Rheumatoid arthritis
- Parapneumonic effusion/empyema
- Churg-Strauss syndrome
- Paragonimiasis

Amylase

Increased pleural fluid amylase levels are seen in patients with malignancy, esophageal rupture, and pancreatic disease.

pH

Causes of pleural effusion with pH <7.20 include:

- Urinothorax
- Paragonimiasis
- Complicated parapneumonic effusion/empyema
- Esophageal rupture
- Tuberculous pleural effusion
- Hemothorax

- Malignancy
- Systemic acidosis
- SLE-associated pleural effusion
- Rheumatoid arthritis

Microbiologic Studies

Pleural fluid may be sent for bacterial, fungal, and mycobacterial culture. For bacteria, aerobic and anaerobic cultures at the bedside are recommended. Patients suspected of having a parapneumonic effusion or empyema should have Gram stain of the pleural fluid in addition to culture. Acid-fast smears of the pleural fluid may be obtained in patients suspected of having tuberculous pleuritis; the yield, however, is low unless the patient has tuberculous empyema.

Cytology

Cytology is positive in 40% to 87% of cases of malignant pleural effusion. The yield varies depending upon a number of factors including number of specimens submitted, mechanism of malignancy, skill of cytologist, type of malignancy, and extent of tumor.

PLEURAL EFFUSIONS

Distinguishing Transudative From Exudative

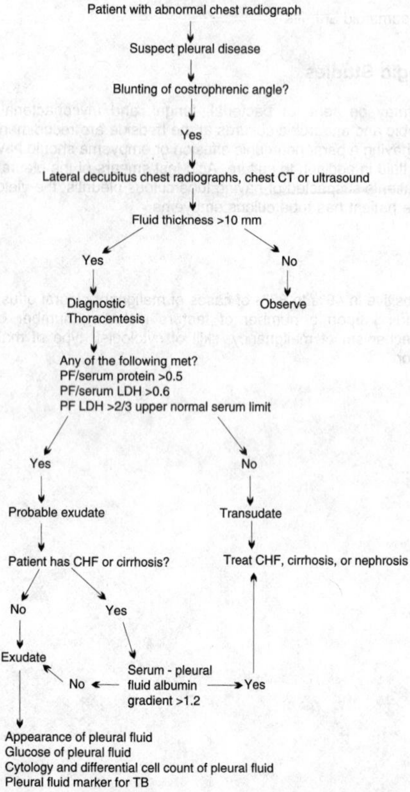
Patient with abnormal chest radiograph
Suspect pleural disease
Blunting of costrophrenic angle?
Yes
Lateral decubitus chest radiographs, chest CT or ultrasound
Fluid thickness >10 mm
Yes
No
Diagnostic Thoracentesis
Observe
Any of the following met?
PF/serum protein >0.5
PF/serum LDH >0.6
PF LDH >2/3 upper normal serum limit
Yes
No
Probable exudate
Transudate
Patient has CHF or cirrhosis?
Treat CHF, cirrhosis, or nephrosis
No
Yes
Exudate
Serum - pleural fluid albumin gradient >1.2
No
Yes
Appearance of pleural fluid
Glucose of pleural fluid
Cytology and differential cell count of pleural fluid
Pleural fluid marker for TB

Adapted from Light R, *Pleural Diseases*, 4th ed, Philadelphia, PA: Lippincott Williams & Wilkins, 2001, 89.

PLEURAL EFFUSIONS

Evaluating the Appearance

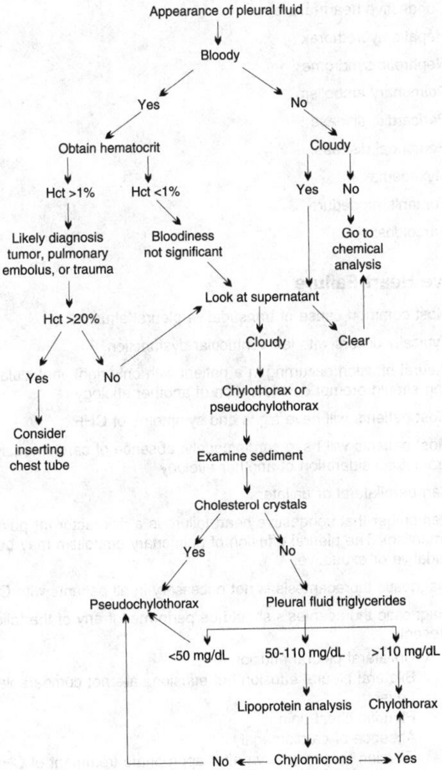
Appearance of pleural fluid
Bloody
Yes
No
Obtain hematocrit
Cloudy
Hct >1%
Hct <1%
Yes
No
Likely diagnosis tumor, pulmonary embolus, or trauma
Bloodiness not significant
Go to chemical analysis
Look at supernatant
Hct >20%
Cloudy
Clear
Yes
No
Chylothorax or pseudochylothorax
Consider inserting chest tube
Examine sediment
Cholesterol crystals
Yes
No
Pseudochylothorax
Pleural fluid triglycerides
<50 mg/dL
50-110 mg/dL
>110 mg/dL
Lipoprotein analysis
Chylothorax
No
Chylomicrons
Yes

Adapted from Light R, *Pleural Diseases*, 4th ed, Philadelphia, PA: Lippincott Williams & Wilkins, 2001, 90.

TRANSUDATIVE PLEURAL EFFUSIONS

Causes of Transudative Pleural Effusion

- Congestive heart failure
- Hepatic hydrothorax
- Nephrotic syndrome
- Pulmonary embolism
- Pericardial disease
- Peritoneal disease
- Myxedema
- Fontan's procedure
- Sarcoidosis

Congestive Heart Failure

- Most common cause of transudative pleural effusion
- Typically occurs with left ventricular dysfunction
- Pleural effusion occurring in a patient with only right ventricular dysfunction should prompt consideration of another etiology
- Most patients will have signs and symptoms of CHF
- Most patients will have cardiomegaly; absence of cardiomegaly should prompt consideration of another etiology
- Can be bilateral or unilateral
- Remember that congestive heart failure is a risk factor for pulmonary embolism. The pleural effusion of pulmonary embolism may be transudative or exudative.
- Diagnostic thoracentesis is not necessary in all patients with CHF
- Diagnostic thoracentesis should be performed if any of the following are present:
  - Unilateral pleural effusion
  - Bilateral pleural effusion but effusions are not comparable in size
  - Fever
  - Pleuritic chest pain
  - Absence of cardiomegaly
  - Effusion fails to resolve after appropriate treatment of CHF

Hepatic Hydrothorax

- Consider in every cirrhotic patient who presents with pleural effusion

- Incidence of hepatic hydrothorax increased in cirrhotic patients who have ascites
- Can be unilateral or bilateral
- Does have a predilection to be right-sided (85%)
- Spontaneous bacterial pleuritis (also known as spontaneous bacterial empyema) is a complication of hepatic hydrothorax. Suspect this diagnosis in patients with hepatic hydrothorax who develop fever. If suspected, obtain pleural fluid culture and neutrophil count.

Nephrotic Syndrome

- Diagnostic thoracentesis is warranted in all patients
- Remember that nephrotic syndrome patients are predisposed to pulmonary embolism. The pleural effusion of pulmonary embolism may be transudative or exudative. Some experts recommend obtaining ventilation/perfusion scan or spiral CT in all patients with nephrotic syndrome who have a transudative pleural effusion.

Pulmonary Embolism

- Effusion tends to be small
- Usually unilateral
- Effusion can be transudative or exudative
- Pleural fluid analysis does not allow diagnosis to be established but is important in excluding other causes of pleural effusion
- If clinical presentation is consistent with pulmonary embolism or no other etiology is found for the effusion, evaluation for pulmonary embolism is warranted.
- Ventilation/perfusion scan is difficult to interpret in patients with pulmonary embolism who present with pleural effusion; yield of the scan may be improved if therapeutic thoracentesis is performed prior to the scan.
- Spiral CT and ultrasound of the leg veins are alternatives to ventilation/perfusion scan.
- When ventilation/perfusion scan, spiral CT, and ultrasound are equivocal or unrevealing in a patient thought to have pleural effusion due to pulmonary embolism, consider pulmonary angiography.

EXUDATIVE PLEURAL EFFUSIONS

Causes of Exudative Pleural Effusion

- Malignancy
  - Metastatic pleural disease
  - Mesothelioma
  - Body cavity lymphoma
- Pulmonary embolism
- Gastrointestinal disease
  - Acute pancreatitis
  - Chronic pancreatitis
  - Intra-abdominal abscess
  - Bilious pleural effusion
  - Diaphragmatic hernia
  - Liver transplantation
  - Postabdominal surgery
  - Endoscopic variceal sclerotherapy
- Postcardiac injury syndrome
- Hemothorax
- Chylothorax
- Drug-induced pleural disease
  - Nitrofurantoin
  - Dantrolene
  - Methysergide
  - Bromocriptine
  - Procarbazine
  - Amiodarone
  - Ergot alkaloids
  - Interleukin-2
  - Methotrexate
  - Clozapine
- Connective tissue disease
  - Pleural effusion of rheumatoid arthritis
  - Lupus arthritis

- Churg-Strauss syndrome
- Wegener's granulomatosis
- Immunoblastic lymphadenopathy
- Sjögren's syndrome
- Familial Mediterranean fever

- Infection
  - Bacterial pneumonia
  - Tuberculous pleuritis
  - Viral
  - *Mycoplasma*
  - Actinomycosis
  - Fungal disease
  - Histoplasmosis
  - Coccidioidomycosis
  - Aspergillosis
  - Blastomycosis
  - Cryptococcosis
  - Parasitic disease
  - Paragonimiasis
  - Amebiasis
  - Echinococcosis
  - *Pneumocystis carinii*
- Miscellaneous
  - Uremia
  - Lung transplantation
  - Bone marrow transplantation
  - Asbestos exposure
  - Sarcoidosis
  - Therapeutic radiation exposure
  - Yellow-nail syndrome
  - Extramedullary hematopoiesis
  - Urinary tract obstruction
  - Meig's syndrome
  - Endometriosis

- Ovarian hyperstimulation syndrome
- Iatrogenic
  - Misplaced percutaneously placed catheter
  - Misplaced nasogastric tube
  - Translumbar aortographic examination
- Trapped lung

Adapted from Light R, *Pleural Diseases*, 4th ed, Philadelphia, PA: Lippincott Williams & Wilkins, 2001, 88.

Parapneumonic Effusion / Empyema

- Pleural effusion occurs in 40% to 60% of patients with bacterial pneumonia
- Most of these effusions are clinically insignificant, not requiring thoracentesis, and resolving with appropriate treatment of the bacterial pneumonia
- A minority of patients, however, may develop complicated parapneumonic effusion or empyema. The term "complicated" is used to describe parapneumonic effusions that do not resolve without chest tube placement. Empyema is defined as the presence of gross pus within the pleural space.
- To differentiate uncomplicated from complicated parapneumonic effusion and empyema, diagnostic thoracentesis is required. However, not all patients with parapneumonic effusion require thoracentesis. Whether or not to perform thoracentesis is based upon the amount of free pleural fluid:
  - Perform thoracentesis if the distance between the inside chest wall and outside the lung is >10 mm
  - Thoracentesis is not required if this distance is <10 mm
- If gross pus is obtained, patient has empyema (chest tube required)
- In the absence of gross pus, the following are consistent with a complicated parapneumonic effusion:
  - Gram stain of pleural fluid positive
  - Pleural fluid glucose <40 mg/dL
  - Pleural fluid culture positive
  - Pleural fluid pH <7.0
  - Pleural fluid LDH >3x upper limit of normal for serum
  - Pleural fluid loculated

  Chest tube placement is warranted in many of these patients.

Malignancy

- Three neoplasms account for 75% of malignant pleural effusions: Lung cancer, breast cancer, and lymphoma
- Effusion can vary from small to massive in size
- Characteristics of pleural fluid include:
  - Exudative
  - Bloody or nonbloody
  - Cell count normal or elevated
  - Lymphocytic predominance most common
  - Glucose normal or low
  - pH normal or low
  - Amylase normal or high
- Definitive diagnosis requires demonstration of malignant cells in pleural fluid or pleura itself
- Cytology positive in 40% to 87% depending upon type of malignancy, skill of cytologist, mechanism of malignant pleural effusion, number of specimens submitted, and extent of tumor
- Cytology superior to needle biopsy of pleura
- In recent years, needle biopsy has largely been replaced by thoracoscopy, which establishes the diagnosis in about 90% of patients

Tuberculous Pleural Effusion

- Usually unilateral effusion
- Can vary in size
- Coexisting lung disease only present in about 20% of patients
- Characteristics of pleural fluid include:
  - Exudative
  - Total protein concentration >5 g/dL
  - >50% with lymphocytic predominance
  - Possible PMN predominance if symptoms present <2 weeks
  - Eosinophils >10% argue strongly against diagnosis
  - Mesothelial cells >5% argue strongly against diagnosis
- Definitive diagnosis requires pleural fluid ADA level, interferon-gamma level, acid-fast smear, pleural fluid culture, or pleural biopsy
- Pleural fluid ADA level >70 units/L is consistent with diagnosis. ADA level <40 units/L should prompt consideration of another etiology.
- Pleural fluid interferon-gamma levels >140 pg/mL strongly suggestive of diagnosis

- Yield of acid-fast smears of pleural fluid low in immunocompetent patients. In HIV patients, acid-fast smears positive in about 20% of cases.
- Cultures of pleural fluid positive for *M. tuberculosis* in <40% of patients
- Needle biopsy demonstrating granulomas consistent with diagnosis. Acid-fast smears and cultures of biopsy material should also be obtained. In recent years, needle biopsy has been supplanted, to some extent, by pleural fluid ADA and interferon-gamma levels.

Pulmonary Embolism

- Effusion tends to be small
- Usually unilateral
- Effusion can be transudative or exudative
- Pleural fluid analysis does not allow diagnosis to be established but is important in excluding other causes of pleural effusion
- If clinical presentation is consistent with pulmonary embolism or no other etiology is found for the effusion, evaluation for pulmonary embolism is warranted.
- Ventilation/perfusion scan is difficult to interpret in patients with pulmonary embolism who present with pleural effusion; yield of the scan may be improved if therapeutic thoracentesis is performed prior to the scan.
- Spiral CT and ultrasound of the leg veins are alternatives to ventilation/perfusion scan.
- When ventilation/perfusion scan, spiral CT, and ultrasound are equivocal or unrevealing in a patient thought to have pleural effusion due to pulmonary embolism, consider pulmonary angiography.

NEUROLOGY

CEREBROSPINAL FLUID ANALYSIS

WBC Count

- While the number of white blood cells varies with age, a count >5 WBC/mm^3 is clearly abnormal after the age of 10 weeks. An increased CSF white blood cell count is termed pleocytosis. The causes of pleocytosis are listed in the following box.

CSF PLEOCYTOSIS DIFFERENTIAL DIAGNOSIS
INFECTION Bacterial Viral Tuberculous Fungal Protozoal INTRACRANIAL LESION NEAR THE SUBARACHNOID SPACE Malignancy Abscess Demyelination Infarct Hemorrhage Vasculitis RECENT SEIZURE RADIATION THERAPY INJECTION OF DRUG INTO THE INTRATHECAL SPACE

- The clinician should realize that the cell count may be spuriously low if it is measured 30-60 minutes after the lumbar puncture. Therefore, it is important to transport the specimen to the laboratory as soon as possible.
- While there are both noninfectious and infectious causes of pleocytosis, infection is always a major concern.
- The degree of WBC count elevation cannot be used alone to reliably differentiate among the infectious causes of meningitis although bacterial meningitis tends to present with higher counts than viral meningitis. In fact, some clinicians maintain that a total WBC count >2000/mm^3 is highly predictive of bacterial meningitis.

- The clinician should realize that pleocytosis is not always present in bacterial meningitis. In fact, up to 4% of patients (more likely to be seen with infants, alcoholics, elderly, and immunocompromised patients) may not have an elevated CSF WBC count. If the clinical presentation is consistent with the diagnosis, the absence of pleocytosis should not cause the clinician to discard the diagnosis. In these cases, Gram stain and culture should still be performed.

- The white blood cells normally present in the CSF are mononuclear cells (lymphocytes and monocytes). An occasional neutrophil, however, may be appreciated.

- When evaluating the patient with a suspected CNS infection, the differential count may provide important information:
  - Preponderance of neutrophils → suggests acute bacterial meningitis
  - Preponderance of lymphocytes → suggests nonbacterial infection (viral, tuberculosis, etc)

- In most cases of acute bacterial meningitis, there is neutrophilic predominance with neutrophils exceeding 90% to 95% of the total WBC count. Ten percent of patients, however, will present with lymphocytic predominance. This is more likely to be seen with early infection, infection due to *Listeria monocytogenes*, and when total WBC counts are <1000/ mm^3.

Glucose

- The normal CSF glucose concentration is less than that of the serum. Since the CSF concentration is dependent on the serum glucose level, a serum glucose level should be obtained at the time of the spinal tap.

- This will allow the clinician to calculate the CSF to serum glucose ratio. Normally, this ratio is approximately 0.6. A ratio below this signifies the presence of low CSF glucose levels. If the serum glucose level is not available, then the lower limit of normal for CSF glucose (about 45 mg/dL) can be used.

- The presence of decreased glucose levels in the CSF is known as hypoglycorrhachia

HYPOGLYCORRHACHIA DIFFERENTIAL DIAGNOSIS	
BACTERIAL MENINGITIS	SUBARACHNOID HEMORRHAGE
TUBERCULOUS MENINGITIS	CYSTICERCOSIS
FUNGAL MENINGITIS	*TRICHINELLA* MENINGITIS
CARCINOMATOUS MENINGITIS	SYPHILIS (acute)
SARCOIDOSIS	VIRAL MENINGOENCEPHALITIS*
HYPOGLYCEMIA	

*While infectious meningitis is a major concern in the patient with hypoglycorrhachia, it is important to recognize that viral infections are usually not characterized by a decrease in the CSF glucose level. There are exceptions to this, however, as low glucose concentrations may be appreciated in patients with meningoencephalitis secondary to mumps, enterovirus, lymphocytic choriomeningitis, herpes simplex, and herpes zoster.

- As shown in the box above, low CSF glucose levels are not just seen in infection but also in noninfectious conditions. In patients suspected of having bacterial meningitis, a low CSF glucose level is helpful in differentiating bacterial from viral infection. The clinician should realize that while viral infection classically presents with normal glucose levels, at times, levels may be low. In addition, not all patients with acute bacterial meningitis will have low CSF glucose concentrations.

Protein

- The upper limit of normal for the CSF protein concentration is about 40-50 mg/dL.
- An increased protein concentration is a nonspecific finding, appreciated in many conditions (both infectious and noninfectious).
- In most patients with acute bacterial meningitis, the concentration exceeds 100 mg/dL. While many patients with viral meningitis have normal protein levels, in some, there is an elevation.
- Some clinicians maintain that a CSF protein concentration >220 mg/dL provides strong evidence for the presence of bacterial infection in patients suspected of having infectious meningitis. It should be noted, however, that some patients with acute bacterial meningitis have normal CSF protein concentrations.

Gram Stain / Culture

- CSF Gram stain and culture should be obtained in every patient in whom bacterial meningitis is a consideration.

- If possible, Gram stain and culture should be obtained before starting the patient on antibiotic therapy.

- Even if the patient has already been started on antibiotic therapy, these studies should still be obtained. Even if the tests are negative, the clinician can often differentiate bacterial from other causes of meningitis based on the rest of the CSF profile (ie, WBC count, differential, protein, glucose).

TYPICAL FINDINGS IN THE CSF OF PATIENTS WITH BACTERIAL MENINGITIS AND ASEPTIC MENINGITIS*

Parameter	Bacterial Meningitis	Aseptic Meningitis†
Opening pressure	>180 mm water	<180 mm water
CSF WBC count	>1000 mm^3	100-1000 mm^3
% neutrophils	>80%	<20%‡
Protein concentration	>100 mg/dL	50-100 mg/dL
Glucose concentration	<40 mg/dL	Normal
CSF / serum glucose ratio	<0.6	>0.6
Gram stain	Positive (about 70%)§	Negative
Culture	Positive (70% to 90%)§	Negative

*CSF tests obtained very early in the course of bacterial meningitis may mimic that found in aseptic meningitis.

†Aseptic meningitis is defined as meningitis presenting with CSF lymphocytic pleocytosis in the setting of unremarkable Gram stain and bacterial cultures of the CSF.

‡May be higher very early in the course.

§Pretreatment with antibiotics is the most important reason for negative result.

From *Clinical Infectious Diseases*, Root RK, ed, New York, NY: Oxford University Press, 1999, 693.

NEPHROLOGY

ACUTE RENAL FAILURE

Although a consensus definition for acute renal failure is lacking, it is characterized by worsening renal function, occurring over hours to days. The decline in renal function leads to the accumulation of nitrogenous waste products, which is reflected as an increase in the serum BUN and creatinine.

Differentiating Acute From Chronic Renal Failure

- Before embarking on a search for the etiology of acute renal failure, the clinician should ensure that the patient has acute rather than chronic renal failure.
- Clinical and laboratory features favoring acute renal failure include:
  - Recent BUN and creatinine levels have been normal
  - Ultrasound reveals normal kidney size
  - Absence of anemia
  - Absence of broad casts in the urine sediment
- Clinical and laboratory features favoring chronic renal failure include:
  - Previous BUN and creatinine levels have been elevated and there is no significant change between the previous and current serum BUN and creatinine levels
  - Ultrasound reveals bilaterally small kidneys
  - Bone radiographs reveal renal osteodystrophy
  - Anemia of chronic renal insufficiency is present
  - Broad casts are found in the urine sediment

Classification of Acute Renal Failure

- Once the presence of acute renal failure has been established, the clinician should perform a thorough history and physical examination along with appropriate laboratory studies to determine the type of acute renal failure present.
- Patients with acute renal failure can be classified into one of the following three groups:
  - Prerenal azotemia
  - Postrenal azotemia
  - Renal azotemia

Postrenal Azotemia

- Postrenal azotemia is defined as acute renal failure resulting from a structural or functional impediment of urine flow, affecting any portion of the urinary tract from the tubules to the urethra.
- Postrenal azotemia accounts for 5% of acute renal failure cases.
- Helpful in establishing the presence of postrenal azotemia are the placement of a Foley catheter and renal ultrasound.
- Placement of a Foley catheter will allow the clinician to measure the postvoid residual. If a large amount of residual urine (>100 mL) is obtained, a lower urinary tract obstruction is the likely cause of the acute renal failure.
- The absence of a large postvoid residual does not exclude upper urinary tract obstruction. For this reason, a renal ultrasound should be performed in most patients with acute renal failure.
- Characteristic ultrasound finding of postrenal azotemia is dilatation of the urinary tract.
- Other tests that may also be helpful include CT scan, intravenous pyelography, and retrograde pyelography (azotemia may, however, be worsened if radiocontrast is administered).

Differentiating Prerenal Azotemia From Renal Azotemia

- Prerenal azotemia is defined as acute renal failure secondary to a decrease in renal perfusion while renal azotemia refers to acute renal failure resulting from disease affecting the renal vasculature, glomeruli, tubules, or interstitium.
- Prerenal azotemia accounts for 55% of acute renal failure cases while renal azotemia accounts for 40% of acute renal failure cases.
- The history and physical examination in combination with appropriate laboratory tests is usually sufficient to differentiate prerenal from renal azotemia. Laboratory tests that should be obtained include the following:
  - Serum BUN and creatinine (to calculate BUN:creatinine ratio)
  - Urine osmolality
  - Fractional excretion of sodium
  - Urine sodium
  - Urinalysis with urine microscopic examination
- BUN:creatinine ratio
  - Ratio >20: Very suggestive of prerenal azotemia
  - Ratio between 10 and 20: Renal azotemia
- Urine osmolality
  - Urine osmolality >500 mOsm/kg: Prerenal azotemia
  - Urine osmolality <350 mOsm/kg: Renal azotemia

- Urine sodium concentration
  - Urine sodium concentration <20 mEq/L: Prerenal azotemia
  - Urine sodium concentration >40 mEq/L: Renal azotemia
- Fractional excretion of sodium (FENa+)
  - Calculation of the fractional excretion of sodium requires sodium and creatinine levels in both urine and plasma
  - FENa+ = (urine sodium x plasma creatinine) / (plasma sodium x urine creatinine) x 100
  - FENa+ <1%: Prerenal azotemia
  - FENa+ >2%: Renal azotemia
  - Some causes of prerenal azotemia are associated with FENa+ >1%. These include diuretic use, bicarbonaturia, pre-existing chronic renal failure complicated by salt wasting, and adrenal insufficiency
  - Some causes of renal azotemia are associated with FENa+ <1%. These include radiocontrast, severe burns, NSAIDs, sepsis, acute glomerulonephritis, vasculitis, and rhabdomyolysis
- Urinalysis with microscopic examination of the urinary sediment should be obtained in every patient presenting with acute renal failure. Findings may include:
  - Unremarkable urinalysis, except for an occasional hyaline cast: Consider prerenal azotemia (postrenal azotemia may also present with normal urinalysis)
  - Positive dipstick for blood but no red blood cells present on microscopic analysis: Consider renal azotemia (hemoglobinuria, myoglobinuria)
  - Hematuria (positive dipstick for blood and red blood cells present on microscopic analysis): Consider renal azotemia (glomerular, tubular, interstitial, or vascular disease) and postrenal azotemia (stones, tumor, blood clots)
  - Red blood cell casts: Consider renal azotemia (glomerular disease, vascular disease, rarely interstitial nephritis)
  - Dysmorphic red blood cells: Consider renal azotemia (glomerular disease)
  - White blood cells / white blood cell casts: Consider renal azotemia (pyelonephritis, interstitial disease)
  - Eosinophiluria (>5%): Consider allergic interstitial nephritis and atheroembolic disease
  - Renal tubular epithelial cells / pigmented casts: Consider renal azotemia (acute tubular necrosis, myoglobinuria, hemoglobinuria

Causes of Prerenal Azotemia

Absolute Decrease in Effective Blood Volume

- Hemorrhage
- Dehydration
- Burns
- Renal loss of fluid
  - Diuretics
  - Osmotic diuretics
  - Adrenal insufficiency
- Third space sequestration
  - Peritonitis
  - Pancreatitis
  - Muscle-crush injury
  - Hypoalbuminemia
- Gastrointestinal fluid loss
  - Vomiting
  - Diarrhea
  - Nasogastric suction

Ineffective Blood Volume

- Decreased cardiac output
- Systemic vasodilation
  - Sepsis
  - Anaphylaxis
  - Anesthesia
  - Antihypertensive therapy
  - Liver failure
- Renal vasoconstriction
  - Hypercalcemia
  - Amphotericin B
  - Cyclosporine
  - Norepinephrine
  - Sepsis
  - Liver disease

Others

- NSAIDs
- ACE inhibitors

ACUTE RENAL FAILURE

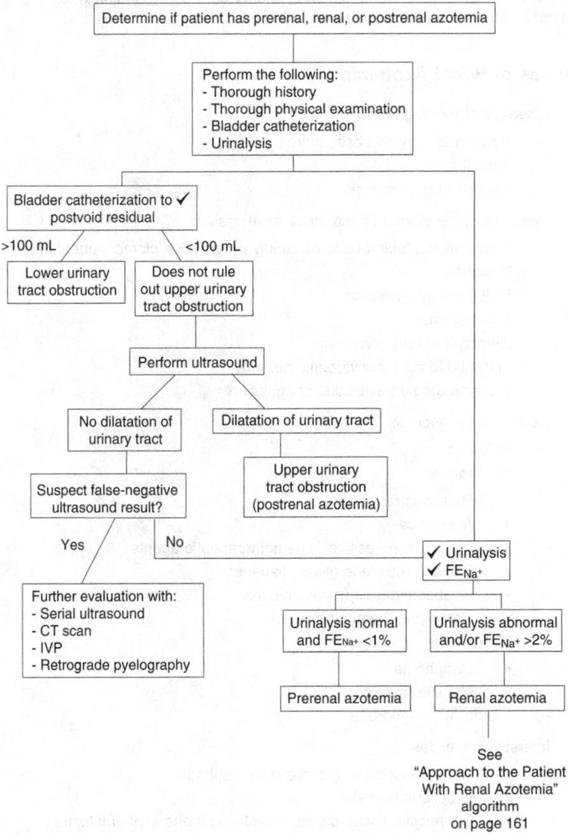
Determine if patient has prerenal, renal, or postrenal azotemia
Perform the following:
- Thorough history
- Thorough physical examination
- Bladder catheterization
- Urinalysis
Bladder catheterization to ✓ postvoid residual
>100 mL
<100 mL
Lower urinary tract obstruction
Does not rule out upper urinary tract obstruction
Perform ultrasound
No dilatation of urinary tract
Dilatation of urinary tract
Upper urinary tract obstruction (postrenal azotemia)
Suspect false-negative ultrasound result?
Yes
No
Further evaluation with:
- Serial ultrasound
- CT scan
- IVP
- Retrograde pyelography
✓ Urinalysis
✓ FENa+
Urinalysis normal and FENa+ <1%
Urinalysis abnormal and/or FENa+ >2%
Prerenal azotemia
Renal azotemia
See "Approach to the Patient With Renal Azotemia" algorithm on page 161

APPROACH TO THE PATIENT WITH RENAL AZOTEMIA

Acute renal failure due to renal azotemia should be a consideration when prerenal and postrenal azotemia have been excluded.

Causes of Renal Azotemia

- Diseases of the large renal vessels
  - Renal artery / vein obstruction
  - Vasculitis
  - Atheroembolic disease
- Diseases of the glomeruli and small renal vessels
  - Glomerulonephritis (acute or rapidly progressive glomerulonephritis)
  - Vasculitis
  - Malignant hypertension
  - Scleroderma
  - Hemolytic-uremic syndrome
  - Thrombotic thrombocytopenic purpura
  - Disseminated intravascular coagulation
- Acute tubular necrosis
  - Ischemic
  - Nephrotoxic
    - Radiocontrast
    - Antibiotics
    - Immunosuppressive / chemotherapeutic agents
    - Poisons (ethylene glycol, toluene)
    - Rhabdomyolysis (myoglobinuria)
    - Hemolysis (hemoglobinuria)
  - Malignancy
    - Lymphoma
    - Multiple myeloma
  - Tumor lysis syndrome
- Interstitial diseases
  - Drug-induced allergic interstitial nephritis
  - Infectious nephritis
  - Connective tissue disease (systemic lupus erythematosus, Sjögren's syndrome)
  - Infiltrative nephritis (hematologic or solid malignancy)

APPROACH TO THE PATIENT WITH RENAL AZOTEMIA

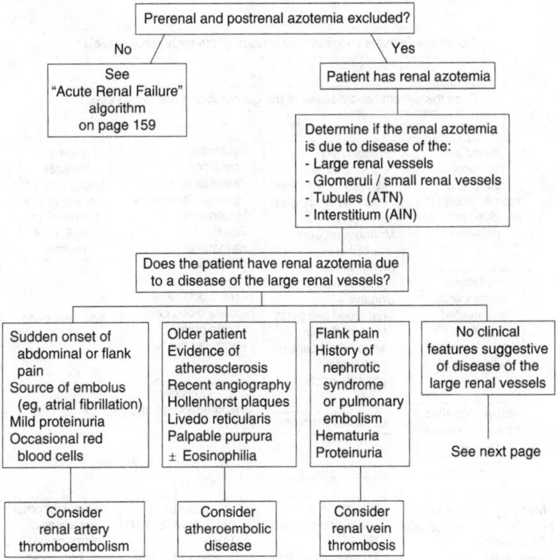
Prerenal and postrenal azotemia excluded?
No
Yes
See "Acute Renal Failure" algorithm on page 159
Patient has renal azotemia
Determine if the renal azotemia is due to disease of the:
- Large renal vessels
- Glomeruli / small renal vessels
- Tubules (ATN)
- Interstitium (AIN)
Does the patient have renal azotemia due to a disease of the large renal vessels?
Sudden onset of abdominal or flank pain
Source of embolus (eg, atrial fibrillation)
Mild proteinuria
Occasional red blood cells
Older patient
Evidence of atherosclerosis
Recent angiography
Hollenhorst plaques
Livedo reticularis
Palpable purpura
± Eosinophilia
Flank pain
History of nephrotic syndrome or pulmonary embolism
Hematuria
Proteinuria
No clinical features suggestive of disease of the large renal vessels
See next page
Consider renal artery thromboembolism
Consider atheroembolic disease
Consider renal vein thrombosis

APPROACH TO THE PATIENT WITH RENAL AZOTEMIA *(continued)*

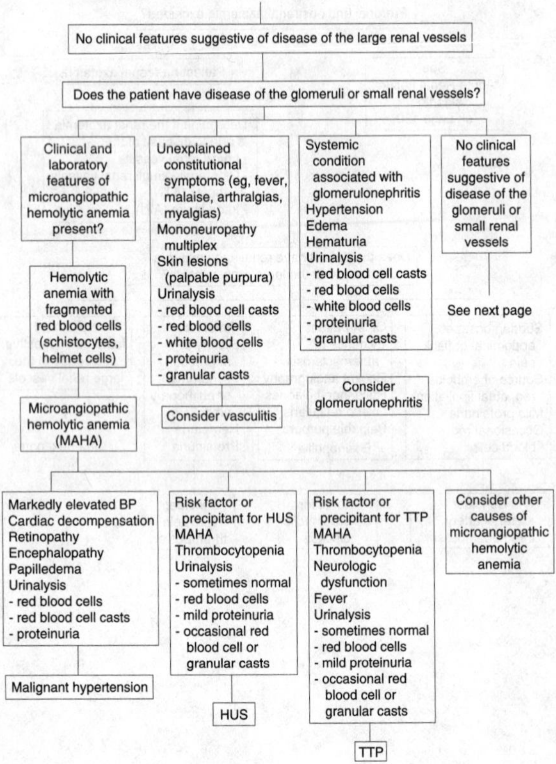
No clinical features suggestive of disease of the large renal vessels
Does the patient have disease of the glomeruli or small renal vessels?
Clinical and laboratory features of microangiopathic hemolytic anemia present?
Hemolytic anemia with fragmented red blood cells (schistocytes, helmet cells)
Microangiopathic hemolytic anemia (MAHA)
Unexplained constitutional symptoms (eg, fever, malaise, arthralgias, myalgias)
Mononeuropathy multiplex
Skin lesions (palpable purpura)
Urinalysis
- red blood cell casts
- red blood cells
- white blood cells
- proteinuria
- granular casts
Consider vasculitis
Systemic condition associated with glomerulonephritis
Hypertension
Edema
Hematuria
Urinalysis
- red blood cell casts
- red blood cells
- white blood cells
- proteinuria
- granular casts
Consider glomerulonephritis
No clinical features suggestive of disease of the glomeruli or small renal vessels
See next page
Markedly elevated BP
Cardiac decompensation
Retinopathy
Encephalopathy
Papilledema
Urinalysis
- red blood cells
- red blood cell casts
- proteinuria
Malignant hypertension
Risk factor or precipitant for HUS
MAHA
Thrombocytopenia
Urinalysis
- sometimes normal
- red blood cells
- mild proteinuria
- occasional red blood cell or granular casts
HUS
Risk factor or precipitant for TTP
MAHA
Thrombocytopenia
Neurologic dysfunction
Fever
Urinalysis
- sometimes normal
- red blood cells
- mild proteinuria
- occasional red blood cell or granular casts
TTP
Consider other causes of microangiopathic hemolytic anemia

APPROACH TO THE PATIENT WITH RENAL AZOTEMIA *(continued)*

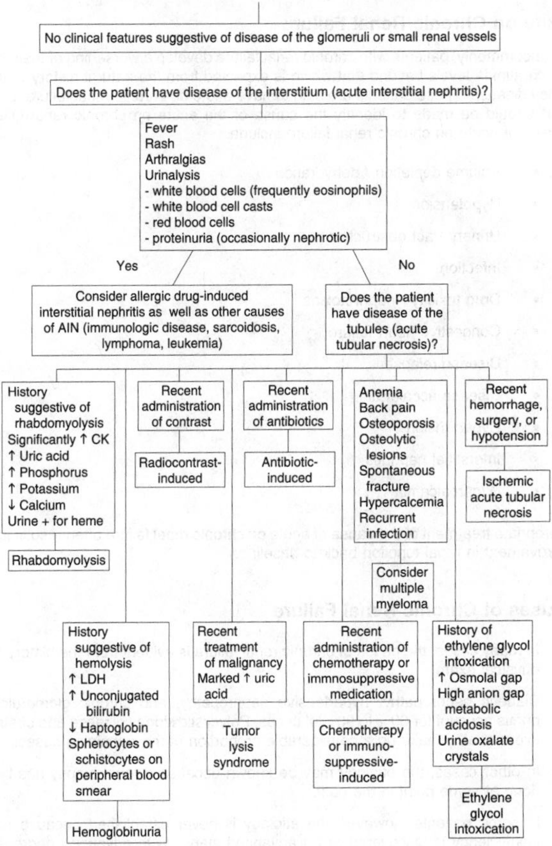
No clinical features suggestive of disease of the glomeruli or small renal vessels
Does the patient have disease of the interstitium (acute interstitial nephritis)?
Fever
Rash
Arthralgias
Urinalysis
- white blood cells (frequently eosinophils)
- white blood cell casts
- red blood cells
- proteinuria (occasionally nephrotic)
Yes
No
Consider allergic drug-induced interstitial nephritis as well as other causes of AIN (immunologic disease, sarcoidosis, lymphoma, leukemia)
Does the patient have disease of the tubules (acute tubular necrosis)?
History suggestive of rhabdomyolysis
Significantly ↑ CK
↑ Uric acid
↑ Phosphorus
↑ Potassium
↓ Calcium
Urine + for heme
Rhabdomyolysis
Recent administration of contrast
Radiocontrast-induced
Recent administration of antibiotics
Antibiotic-induced
Anemia
Back pain
Osteoporosis
Osteolytic lesions
Spontaneous fracture
Hypercalcemia
Recurrent infection
Consider multiple myeloma
Recent hemorrhage, surgery, or hypotension
Ischemic acute tubular necrosis
History suggestive of hemolysis
↑ LDH
↑ Unconjugated bilirubin
↓ Haptoglobin
Spherocytes or schistocytes on peripheral blood smear
Hemoglobinuria
Recent treatment of malignancy
Marked ↑ uric acid
Tumor lysis syndrome
Recent administration of chemotherapy or immnosuppressive medication
Chemotherapy or immuno-suppressive-induced
History of ethylene glycol intoxication
↑ Osmolal gap
High anion gap metabolic acidosis
Urine oxalate crystals
Ethylene glycol intoxication

CHRONIC RENAL FAILURE

Acute on Chronic Renal Failure

Not uncommonly, patients with chronic renal failure develop a worsening of their BUN and creatinine levels beyond that which is expected from the natural history of their kidney disease. These patients are said to have acute on chronic renal failure. Every effort should be made to identify the cause of the acute on chronic renal failure. Causes of acute on chronic renal failure include:

- Volume depletion / dehydration
- Hypotension
- Urinary tract obstruction
- Infection
- Drug toxicity / nephrotoxins
- Congestive heart failure
- Disease relapse
- Disease acceleration
- Hypertension
- Interstitial nephritis
- Hypercalcemia

Appropriate treatment of the cause of acute on chronic renal failure often results in an improvement in renal function back to baseline.

Causes of Chronic Renal Failure

- In many cases, the cause of chronic renal failure is evident from the history and physical exam.
- Diabetic nephropathy, hypertensive nephropathy, and chronic glomerulonephritis account for 60% to 90% of cases. Polycystic kidney disease and obstructive uropathy make up a considerable proportion of the remaining cases.
- In other cases, the etiology may be known because a renal biopsy has been done at some point in the past.
- In some patients, however, the etiology is never established because renal insufficiency is discovered at an advanced stage. With advanced degrees of renal dysfunction, biopsy is often not done because of the low probability of finding a reversible lesion.

Laboratory Test Findings in Chronic Renal Failure

- Laboratory testing that may help elucidate the etiology of the chronic renal failure includes the following:
  - Heavy proteinuria (>3.5 g/day): Glomerular disease
  - Mild proteinuria (<1.5 g/day): Tubulointerstitial disease
  - Urine RBC casts: Glomerular disease
  - Urine WBC casts: Tubulointerstitial disease
  - + SPEP / UPEP: Multiple myeloma, light chain deposition disease
  - + ANA: Systemic lupus erythematosus
  - + ANCA: Wegener's granulomatosis, other small vessel vasculitis
  - Hypocomplementemia: Systemic lupus erythematosus, membranoproliferative glomerulonephritis
  - Hypercalcemia: Hypercalcemia-induced nephropathy
- Other laboratory test abnormalities that may be appreciated in chronic renal failure patients include the following:
  - Hypocalcemia
  - Hyperphosphatemia
  - Hyperkalemia
  - Metabolic acidosis
  - Hyperuricemia
  - Increased PTH
  - Anemia (typically normocytic, normochromic)
  - Hypertriglyceridemia

Estimating the Severity of the Chronic Renal Failure

The severity of the chronic renal failure may be estimated by calculating the creatinine clearance. This calculation, however, requires performing a 24-hour urine collection. Many patients find the 24-hour urine collection cumbersome. Because an inadequate collection can lead to an inaccurate estimation of the severity of chronic renal failure, many clinicians rely on the Cockcroft-Gault formula for the calculation of the creatinine clearance:

$$\textbf{Creatinine clearance} = \frac{[(140 - \text{age}) \times \text{wt (kg)}]}{(72 \times \text{serum creatinine})}$$

For women, multiply the result by 0.85

When the creatinine clearance falls below 20 mL/minute, the clinician should discuss issues regarding renal replacement therapy (ie, dialysis).

NEPHROTIC SYNDROME

FEATURES OF THE NEPHROTIC SYNDROME
NEPHROTIC RANGE PROTEINURIA (>3.5 g/1.73 m^2 in 24 hours)
HYPOALBUMINEMIA
HYPERLIPIDEMIA
EDEMA
LIPIDURIA
Fat droplets
Oval fat bodies
Fatty / waxy casts

Major Causes of the Nephrotic Syndrome

- Primary renal disease
  - Membranous nephropathy
  - Focal glomerulosclerosis
  - IgA nephropathy
  - Minimal change disease
  - Membranoproliferative glomerulonephritis
  - Other
- Systemic diseases
  - Diabetes mellitus
  - Amyloidosis
  - Systemic lupus erythematosus
  - Dysproteinemia
    - Multiple myeloma
    - Immunotactoid / fibrillary glomerulonephritis
    - Light chain deposition disease
    - Heavy chain deposition disease
  - Infection
    - Human immunodeficiency virus
    - Hepatitis B
    - Hepatitis C
    - Syphilis

    - Schistosomiasis
    - Tuberculosis
    - Leprosy
  - Malignancy
    - Solid adenocarcinomas (eg, lung, breast, colon)
    - Hodgkin's lymphoma
    - Other malignant neoplasms
  - Drugs or toxins
    - NSAIDs
    - Gold
    - Penicillamine
    - Probenecid
    - Mercury
    - Captopril
    - Heroin
  - Other
    - Pre-eclampsia
    - Chronic allograft rejection
    - Vesicoureteral reflux
    - Bee sting

Adapted from Madaio MP and Harrington JT, "The Diagnosis of Glomerular Diseases," *Arch Intern Med*, 2001, 161:30.

Establishing the Etiology of the Nephrotic Syndrome

Of key importance is the performance of a thorough history and physical examination to assess for the presence of systemic causes of the nephrotic syndrome. The evaluation of the nephrotic syndrome in adults should include the following:

- History
  - Family history and history of drug or toxin exposure
- Physical examination
  - If patient is >50 years, usual recommendations for age, including stool examination (hemoccult testing 3x)
    - If stool examination is negative, perform flexible sigmoidoscopy
    - If stool examination is positive, perform standard GI tract work-up
- Laboratory testing
  - CBC

- Serum BUN
- Serum creatinine
- Glucose
- AST
- ALT
- LDH
- Alkaline phosphatase
- Albumin
- Lipid profile
- Chest radiograph

- Consider systemic diseases
  - Fluorescein angiography (for diabetes mellitus)
  - Antinuclear antibodies (for systemic lupus erythematosus)
- Consider malignant neoplasm (eg, amyloid or light chain deposition disease or myeloma)
  - If patient is >50 years or initial evaluation raises suspicion, perform:
    - Serum protein electrophoresis
    - Serum immunoelectrophoresis
    - Urine protein electrophoresis
    - Abdominal fat-pad biopsy
- Consider infection
  - Perform the following:
    - Hepatitis B serology
    - Hepatitis C serology
    - HIV testing
- Renal biopsy
  - Distinguish primary glomerular disease
  - Diagnosis of unsuspected secondary glomerular disease (eg, amyloid)
  - Determine disease severity

Adapted from Madaio MP and Harrington JT, "The Diagnosis of Glomerular Diseases," *Arch Intern Med*, 2001, 161:32

ACUTE GLOMERULONEPHRITIS

Features of Acute Glomerulonephritis

- Hematuria
- Red blood cell casts
- Proteinuria (usually non-nephrotic range)
- Oliguria
- Acute renal failure
- Hypertension
- Edema

Major Causes of Acute Glomerulonephritis

- Systemic disease
  - Systemic lupus erythematosus
  - Cryoglobulinemia
  - Subacute bacterial endocarditis
  - Shunt nephritis
  - Polyarteritis nodosa
  - Wegener's granulomatosis
  - Hypersensitivity vasculitis
  - Henöch-Schonlein purpura
  - Goodpasture's syndrome
  - Visceral abscess
- Renal disease
  - Acute poststreptococcal glomerulonephritis
  - Membranoproliferative glomerulonephritis
  - IgA nephropathy
  - Idiopathic rapidly progressive glomerulonephritis
    - Anti-GBM disease
    - Pauci-immune disease
    - Immune-deposit disease

Serologic Testing Recommended in Patients With Acute Glomerulonephritis

- In some cases, clues present in the history and physical exam may point to a particular etiology. In these cases, the appropriate laboratory testing and studies should be performed to confirm the diagnosis.
- In other cases, the etiology is not clear. In these cases, the following serologic tests are recommended:
  - Complement levels (C3, C5, CH50)
  - Anti-DNA antibodies

- ANCA
- Cryoglobulins
- Hepatitis B serology
- Hepatitis C serology
- Blood cultures
- Anti-GBM antibodies
- Streptozyme

Serum Complement Levels in the Major Causes of Acute Glomerulonephritis

- Particularly useful in the evaluation of these patients are complement levels.
- Hypocomplementemia should prompt consideration of the following causes of acute glomerulonephritis:
  - Systemic lupus erythematosus
  - Cryoglobulinemia
  - Subacute bacterial endocarditis
  - Shunt nephritis
  - Acute poststreptococcal glomerulonephritis
  - Membranoproliferative glomerulonephritis (type I and II)
- Normocomplementemia should prompt consideration of the following causes of acute glomerulonephritis:
  - Polyarteritis nodosa
  - Wegener's granulomatosis
  - Hypersensitivity vasculitis
  - Henöch-Schonlein purpura
  - Goodpasture's syndrome
  - Visceral abscess
  - IgA nephropathy
  - Idiopathic rapidly progressive (anti-GBM disease, pauci-immune, immune-deposit disease)

HEMATURIA

Hematuria is defined as the presence of blood in the urine. It may be either gross or microscopic. When hematuria is gross, it causes concern in both patients and clinicians alike. In particular, there is concern that the hematuria may be caused by a serious condition (ie, malignancy). It is important to realize, however, that the causes of gross and microscopic hematuria are essentially the same. Therefore, a thorough evaluation is necessary in all patients with hematuria irrespective of whether it is microscopic or gross.

Establishing the Presence of Hematuria

A positive urine dipstick for blood is usually noted in both gross and microscopic hematuria. However, a positive urine dipstick test result is not synonymous with hematuria. Causes of a positive urine dipstick for blood include the following:

- Hematuria
- Hemoglobinuria
- Myoglobinuria

To differentiate among the above causes of a positive urine dipstick for blood, the clinician should perform urine microscopy. Hematuria is present when microscopic examination of the urine reveals >3 red blood cells per high power field. The absence of red blood cells should prompt consideration of hemoglobinuria or myoglobinuria.

Causes of Hematuria

INTRARENAL

- Glomerular
  - Primary
    - Alport's syndrome
    - Focal segmental glomerulosclerosis
    - IgA nephropathy
    - Membranous nephropathy
    - Membranous glomerulonephritis
    - Minimal change disease
    - Rapidly progressive glomerulonephritis
    - Thin basement membrane disease

  - Secondary
    - Anti-GBM disease
    - Hemolytic-uremic syndrome
    - Henöch-Schonlein purpura
    - Mixed essential cryoglobulinemia
    - Postinfectious glomerulonephritis
    - Systemic lupus erythematosus
    - Vasculitis
- Nonglomerular
  - Familial
    - Medullary cystic or sponge kidney
    - Polycystic kidney disease
  - Hydronephrosis
  - Malignancy
  - Metabolic
    - Hyperuricosuria
    - Hypercalciuria
  - Papillary necrosis
    - Analgesic abuse
    - Diabetes mellitus
    - Obstructive uropathy
    - Sickle cell disease or trait
  - Trauma
  - Vascular
    - Malignant hypertension
    - Renal infarct
    - Renal vein thrombosis

EXTRARENAL

- Bleeding disorder
- Infection
  - Cystitis
  - Prostatitis
  - Schistosomiasis
  - Tuberculosis
  - Urethritis

- Malignancy
  - Prostate adenocarcinoma
  - Transitional cell cancer of the urinary tract
- Medications
  - Anticoagulants
  - Cyclophosphamide
- Stones
- Trauma

Differentiating Glomerular From Nonglomerular Hematuria

The differential diagnosis of hematuria can be narrowed considerably by determining if the patient has glomerular or nonglomerular bleeding:

- Characteristics of glomerular bleeding:
  - Red blood cell casts often present
  - Dysmorphic red blood cells often present
  - Absence of blood clots in urine
  - Protein excretion usually >500 mg/day
- Characteristics of nonglomerular bleeding:
  - Red blood cell casts absent
  - Dysmorphic red blood cells absent
  - Blood clots in urine may be present
  - Protein excretion usually <500 mg/day

Evaluation of Glomerular Hematuria

Laboratory testing that may help elucidate the etiology of the glomerular bleeding includes the following:

- Hypocomplementemia: Systemic lupus erythematosus, cryoglobulinemia, poststreptococcal glomerulonephritis, postinfectious glomerulonephritis, membranoproliferative glomerulonephritis
- \+ ANA: Systemic lupus erythematosus
- \+ ANCA: Wegener's glomerulonephritis, other small vessel vasculitis
- \+ Anti-GBM: Anti-GBM nephritis, Goodpasture's syndrome
- \+ Cryoglobulins: Cryoglobulinemia
- \+ Anti-HCV: Hepatitis C associated membranoproliferative glomerulonephritis
- \+ Antistreptolysin O: Poststreptococcal glomerulonephritis

If the results of the history, physical examination, and laboratory testing do not elucidate the etiology of the glomerular hematuria, consideration should be given to renal biopsy. Studies have shown that renal biopsy does not alter treatment or prognosis in patients unless they have hypertension, decreased renal function, or proteinuria. Renal biopsy should seriously be considered if one or more of these features are present.

In the absence of these features, patients should be evaluated periodically (BP, serum BUN, serum creatinine, creatinine clearance, 24-hour urine collection for protein). The development of hypertension, renal insufficiency, or worsening proteinuria should prompt referral for renal biopsy.

HEMATURIA

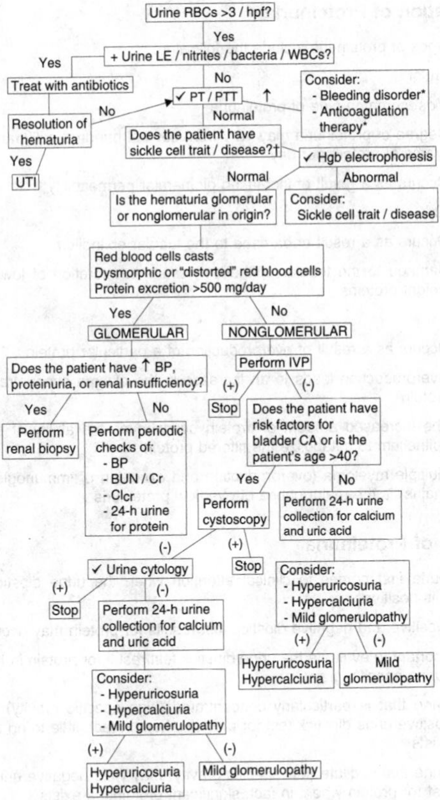
Urine RBCs >3 / hpf?
Yes
+ Urine LE / nitrites / bacteria / WBCs?
Yes
Treat with antibiotics
Resolution of hematuria
Yes
UTI
No
No
✓ PT / PTT
↑
Consider:
- Bleeding disorder*
- Anticoagulation therapy*
Normal
Does the patient have sickle cell trait / disease?†
✓ Hgb electrophoresis
Normal
Abnormal
Is the hematuria glomerular or nonglomerular in origin?
Consider:
Sickle cell trait / disease
Red blood cells casts
Dysmorphic or "distorted" red blood cells
Protein excretion >500 mg/day
Yes
No
GLOMERULAR
NONGLOMERULAR
Does the patient have ↑ BP, proteinuria, or renal insufficiency?
Yes
No
Perform renal biopsy
Perform periodic checks of:
- BP
- BUN / Cr
- Clcr
- 24-h urine for protein
Perform IVP
(+)
(-)
Stop
Does the patient have risk factors for bladder CA or is the patient's age >40?
Yes
No
Perform cystoscopy
Perform 24-h urine collection for calcium and uric acid
(-)
(+)
Stop
✓ Urine cytology
(+)
(-)
Stop
Perform 24-h urine collection for calcium and uric acid
Consider:
- Hyperuricosuria
- Hypercalciuria
- Mild glomerulopathy
(+)
(-)
Hyperuricosuria
Hypercalciuria
Mild glomerulopathy
Consider:
- Hyperuricosuria
- Hypercalciuria
- Mild glomerulopathy
(+)
(-)
Hyperuricosuria
Hypercalciuria
Mild glomerulopathy

*Hematuria that occurs in the patient with an elevated PT / PTT may be the result of anticoagulation therapy or a bleeding disorder. However, an underlying structural etiology cannot be excluded.

†Sickle cell trait/disease may be the sole cause of hematuria; however, this diagnosis must be one of exclusion.

PROTEINURIA

Classification of Proteinuria

The three types of proteinuria include the following:

- Glomerular
  - Most common type of proteinuria
  - Degree of proteinuria may vary from several hundred milligrams to >100 grams of protein per day
  - Occurs as a result of increased glomerular permeability
- Tubular
  - Occurs as a result of damage to the tubular epithelium
  - Damage to the tubular epithelium results in excretion of low molecular weight proteins
- Overflow
  - Occurs as a result of overproduction of a particular protein
  - Overproduction leads to an increase in the plasma concentration of the protein
  - The increased amount of protein overwhelms the ability of the tubular epithelium to catabolize the filtered protein
  - Multiple myeloma (overproduction and excretion of immunoglobulin light chains) is the major cause of overflow proteinuria

Detection of Proteinuria

- Proteinuria first comes to clinical attention when the urine dipstick test for protein is positive
- False-positive and negative dipstick test results for protein may occur
- It is important to evaluate the urine dipstick test result for protein in the context of the urine specific gravity:
  - Urine that is particularly concentrated (high specific gravity) may yield positive urine dipstick test for protein when, in fact, little to no proteinuria exists
  - Urine that is dilute (low specific gravity) may yield negative urine dipstick test for protein when, in fact, significant proteinuria exists
- The urine dipstick test for protein will not be positive in patients who have low molecular weight proteinuria (ie, multiple myeloma). Better test in these patients is the sulfosalicylic acid test or urine protein electrophoresis

24-Hour Urine Collection for Protein

- Urine dipstick test for protein is not a quantitative test for protein but rather a semiquantitative test.
- Therefore, when persistent proteinuria is demonstrated by urine dipstick testing, a 24-hour urine collection for protein should be performed to determine the degree of proteinuria.
- To ensure that the collection is complete, creatinine should also be measured in the 24-hour urine collection:
  - Males excrete 20-25 mg/kg creatinine in a 24-hour period
  - Females excrete 15-20 mg/kg creatinine in a 24-hour period
- Normal protein excretion over a 24-hour time period is <150 mg
- Excretion of >3.5 g/1.73 m^2 in a 24-hour time period is consistent with nephrotic-range proteinuria.

Urine Protein:Creatinine Ratio

- Because the 24-hour urine collection is cumbersome, some prefer to calculate the urine protein:creatinine ratio as a surrogate to the 24-hour urine collection for protein.
- Advantage of the urine protein:creatinine ratio is that it can be done on a random spot urine.
- The ratio is calculated by dividing the urine protein measured in mg/dL by the urine creatinine measured in mg/dL.
- The ratio will correlate to the total amount of protein excreted as determined by the 24-hour urine collection. For example, a urine protein to creatinine ratio of 4 corresponds to the excretion of 4 grams of protein over a 24-hour time period.

Differentiating Glomerular Proteinuria From Tubular / Overflow Proteinuria

- Differential diagnosis of proteinuria can be narrowed considerably by determining if the patient has glomerular, tubular, or overflow proteinuria.
- Glomerular proteinuria is likely if hematuria is present, especially if red blood cell casts or dysmorphic red blood cells are noted on examination of the urinary sediment.
- When hematuria is not present, the 24-hour urine collection for protein or urine protein:creatinine ratio can help differentiate glomerular from tubular / overflow proteinuria:
  - If protein excretion exceeds 3 g/day, glomerular proteinuria is very likely
  - If protein excretion is <3 g/day, glomerular, tubular, or overflow proteinuria may be present

- Urine protein electrophoresis is a useful test in patients who excrete <3 g of protein/day.
  - When albumin represents >70% of the total protein, glomerular proteinuria is said to be present
  - When the excretion of globulins exceeds that of albumin, tubular or overflow proteinuria is said to be present
- To distinguish between tubular and overflow proteinuria, further examination of the urine protein electrophoresis is often helpful:
  - Presence of a single globulin peak is consistent with overflow proteinuria (ie, multiple myeloma)
  - Presence of multiple peaks (representing the excretion of many different globulins) is consistent with tubular proteinuria

PROTEINURIA

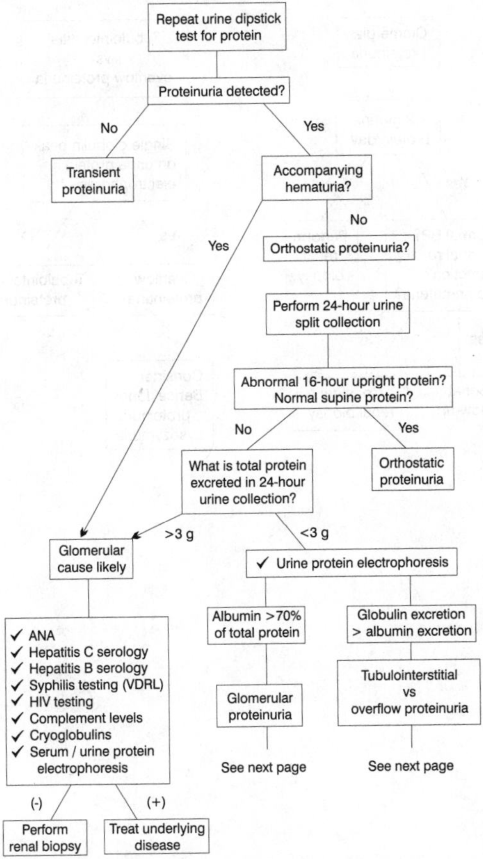
Repeat urine dipstick test for protein
Proteinuria detected?
No
Yes
Transient proteinuria
Accompanying hematuria?
Yes
No
Orthostatic proteinuria?
Perform 24-hour urine split collection
Abnormal 16-hour upright protein? Normal supine protein?
No
Yes
What is total protein excreted in 24-hour urine collection?
Orthostatic proteinuria
>3 g
<3 g
Glomerular cause likely
✓ Urine protein electrophoresis
Albumin >70% of total protein
Globulin excretion > albumin excretion
✓ ANA
✓ Hepatitis C serology
✓ Hepatitis B serology
✓ Syphilis testing (VDRL)
✓ HIV testing
✓ Complement levels
✓ Cryoglobulins
✓ Serum / urine protein electrophoresis
Glomerular proteinuria
Tubulointerstitial vs overflow proteinuria
See next page
See next page
(-)
(+)
Perform renal biopsy
Treat underlying disease

PROTEINURIA (*continued*)

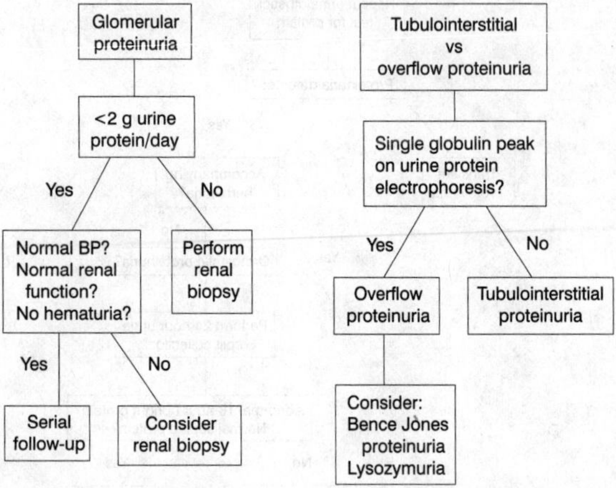
Glomerular proteinuria
<2 g urine protein/day
Yes
No
Normal BP? Normal renal function? No hematuria?
Perform renal biopsy
Yes
No
Serial follow-up
Consider renal biopsy
Tubulointerstitial vs overflow proteinuria
Single globulin peak on urine protein electrophoresis?
Yes
No
Overflow proteinuria
Tubulointerstitial proteinuria
Consider: Bence Jones proteinuria Lysozymuria

MICROALBUMINURIA

- The term "microalbuminuria" is really a misnomer. It does not refer to an abnormal structure of albumin. It really refers to the urinary excretion of albumin that is below the detection capability of the urine dipstick (300-500 mg/day) but above the upper limit of normal for healthy individuals.

- The detection of microalbuminuria is particularly important in diabetic patients because it is the earliest clinical finding of diabetic nephropathy.

- Diabetes mellitus patients should be screened for microalbuminuria:
  - Testing for microalbuminuria should be performed annually in diabetes mellitus type I, beginning 5 years after the diagnosis
  - Testing for microalbuminuria should be performed annually in diabetes mellitus type II, beginning at the time of diagnosis

- 24-hour urine collection is the gold standard for the detection of microalbuminuria.

- Another option is the calculation of the albumin:creatinine ratio on an untimed urine specimen (ratio >30 mg/g is considered a positive test result).

- Fever, exercise, and congestive heart failure are other causes of microalbuminuria; these transient causes of microalbuminuria should be differentiated from those due to diabetes by repeating the test for microalbumin.

PROSTATE-SPECIFIC ANTIGEN (PSA)

Screening for Prostate Cancer

- American Cancer Society and the American Urological Association advocate yearly digital rectal examination and measurement of the serum PSA in asymptomatic men older than the age of 50. Annual screening at the age of 40 years is recommended in high-risk individuals (African-American men, men who have first-degree relatives with prostate cancer).
- The results of the screening PSA level and digital rectal examination can be used to guide further management:
  - Negative digital rectal exam and elevated serum PSA level: Transrectal ultrasonography with biopsy
  - Suspicious digital rectal examination and normal serum PSA level: Transrectal ultrasonography with biopsy
  - Suspicious digital rectal examination and elevated serum PSA level: Transrectal ultrasonography with biopsy
  - Negative digital rectal exam and normal serum PSA level: Annual PSA and digital rectal examination
- Although serum PSA testing is recommended by some organizations for prostate cancer screening, other organizations such as the U.S. Preventive Services Task Force do not recommend the routine use of the PSA as a screening tool for the early detection of prostate cancer.

Sensitivity of PSA in the Detection of Prostate Cancer

- Upper limit of normal for PSA is about 4 ng/mL
- Most prostate cancers are associated with an elevated PSA
- About 20% to 30%, however, will present with a normal PSA level

Specificity of PSA in the Detection of Prostate Cancer

- Any condition that leads to the disruption of the normal architecture of the prostate gland can result in an increase in the serum PSA level
- Specificity for prostate cancer is about 60% to 70% when the serum PSA level is >4 ng/mL
- Causes of serum PSA elevation include the following:
  - Prostate cancer
  - Benign prostatic hyperplasia (BPH)
  - Prostatitis (acute, subclinical, chronic)
  - Prostate infarction
  - Prostatic massage

- Urinary retention
- Physical activity
- Infection
- Medications
- Ejaculation (PSA increase is not clinically significant)
- Digital rectal exam (PSA increase is not clinically significant)
- Prostate biopsy
- Cystoscopy

PSA Modifications

- PSA modifications include age-adjusted PSA, PSA velocity, free:total PSA ratio, and PSA density.
- These modifications to the PSA test have been developed to increase the sensitivity and specificity of the PSA.
- At the current time, there is no consensus regarding the optimal use of these modifications.

Use of PSA Following Radical Prostatectomy

- Undetectable levels following radical prostatectomy suggest that the patient has been cured of prostate cancer.
- Undetectable levels are expected within 1 month of surgery.
- If levels do not become undetectable within 1 month of surgery, then the clinician should suspect residual disease.
- If the serum PSA becomes undetectable within 1 month of surgery only to become detectable during follow-up, then the clinician should suspect disease recurrence.

HYPERURICEMIA

- Hyperuricemia occurs because of increased production of uric acid, decreased excretion of uric acid, or both.
- Hyperuricemia can be primary or secondary.
- Primary hyperuricemia is present if there is no condition causing increased production or decreased excretion of uric acid.
- Secondary hyperuricemia is present if excessive production of uric acid, decreased excretion of uric acid, or both is due to an identifiable condition.
- Causes of secondary hyperuricemia due to excessive production of uric acid:
  - Inherited enzyme defects
  - Myeloproliferative disorders
  - Lymphoproliferative disorders
  - Tissue hypoxia
  - Obesity
  - Malignancy
  - Psoriasis
  - Hemolytic disorders
  - Excessive dietary intake of purines
  - Alcohol
  - Vitamin B_{12}
  - Nicotinic acid
  - Cytotoxic drugs
  - Coumadin®
- Causes of secondary hyperuricemia due to decreased excretion of uric acid
  - Chronic renal failure
  - Lead nephropathy
  - Obesity
  - Volume depletion
  - Lactic acidosis
  - Ketoacidosis (diabetic, starvation)
  - Hypothyroidism
  - Hyperparathyroidism
  - Sarcoidosis
  - Diuretics (thiazide, loop)
  - Low-dose salicylates

- Ethambutol
- Pyrazinamide
- Cyclosporine
- Alcohol
- Levodopa
- Methoxyflurane
- Laxative abuse (alkalosis)

- Once hyperuricemia is identified, every effort should be made to look for underlying disorder or medication associated with hyperuricemia.
- If the history and physical examination does not reveal etiology, a 24-hour urine collection for uric acid should be performed while patient is on a standard diet and free of medications that can interfere with uric acid metabolism.
- Excessive excretion of uric acid is defined as 24-hour urine uric acid >800 mg/day or 12 mg/kg/day.
- The 24-hour urine collection results will help to narrow the differential diagnosis of hyperuricemia and help guide therapy if needed.

URINALYSIS

A complete urinalysis includes chemical analysis of the urine using reagent strips (dipstick testing) and examination of the urine sediment. To perform the urinalysis, urine is centrifuged at 3000 rpm for 3-5 minutes. The supernatant is then separated from the sediment. A small amount of the sediment should be placed on a slide for microscopic examination. When reagent strips are wetted by the supernatant, a chemical reaction takes place, which results in a change of color. The color obtained may be compared to a color chart that is distributed by the manufacturer to give qualitative results for the following tests:

- pH
- Protein
- Glucose
- Ketones
- Bilirubin
- Urobilinogen
- Blood
- Nitrites
- Leukocyte esterase
- Specific gravity

The results may be reported as one of the following, depending upon the type of reagent strips that are used:

- Concentration (mg/dL)
- Small / moderate / large
- 1+/2+/3+/4+
- +/-/normal

Exceptions to this are specific gravity and pH, which are always given a numerical value.

For further discussion, see Urine Dipstick Testing *on page 187.*

Examination of the urine sediment is discussed further *on page 191.*

URINE DIPSTICK TESTING

Color

- Normal color is clear and light yellow.
- Color varies with concentration of the urine (lighter when dilute and darker when concentrated).
- Major causes of white urine color is pyuria and phosphaturia.
- Major causes of green urine color is methylene blue, amitriptyline, and propofol.
- Major causes of black urine color is malignancy and ochronosis.
- Although there are many causes of red or brown urine, major concerns are hematuria, hemoglobinuria, and myoglobinuria.
  - Initial step in the evaluation of red or brown urine is centrifugation of the urine specimen
  - If redness is only present in urine sediment, hematuria is present
  - If redness is present only in the supernatant, the supernatant should be tested for heme by urine dipstick
  - Positive dipstick test result for heme consistent with hemoglobinuria or myoglobinuria
  - Can differentiate between hemoglobinuria and myoglobinuria by looking at the color of plasma (red color of plasma consistent with hemoglobinuria while normal plasma color is consistent with myoglobinuria)

Protein

- Urine dipstick for protein really only tests for the presence of albumin.
- Urine dipstick for protein does not detect other types of proteins as well including immunoglobulin light chains.
  - Sulfosalicylic acid test is better for detecting immunoglobulin light chains
  - Positive sulfosalicylic acid test in the setting of a negative urine dipstick test for protein is suggestive of the presence of nonalbumin proteins (most common scenario is monoclonal gammopathy like multiple myeloma)
- Even with albumin, the urine dipstick test is not very sensitive since protein excretion must be in excess of 300-500 mg/day for the dipstick test result to be positive. Upper limit of normal protein excretion is 150 mg/day.
- This is important especially in patients with diabetes mellitus in whom the earliest clinical finding suggestive of diabetic nephropathy is the excretion of 150-300 mg of protein per day (microalbuminuria). For this reason, diabetic patients are screened with microalbumin tests.

- Urine dipstick test results for protein should always be interpreted in the context of the urine specific gravity:
  - Degree of proteinuria will be underestimated in dilute urine (low specific gravity)
  - Degree of proteinuria will be overestimated in concentrated urine (high specific gravity)
- False-positive test results occur within 24 hours of radiocontrast administration.
- Dipstick testing for protein is not quantitative but semiquantitative (for this reason persistent proteinuria demonstrated by dipstick testing should always be followed up with 24-hour urine collection for protein).

pH

- pH provides information regarding the degree of urine acidification.
- pH varies from 4.5-8.0.
- pH is important in the evaluation of metabolic acidosis.
  - In patients with metabolic acidosis, appropriate response is a decrease in the pH to <5-5.5
  - Failure to decrease to these levels suggests the presence of renal tubular acidosis
- In patients with urinary tract infection, pH >7-7.5 is suggestive of the presence of a urea-splitting organism.

Urine Osmolality

- Urine osmolality is a measure of solute concentration of the urine.
- Urine osmolality is a useful test in the evaluation of patients with hyponatremia, hypernatremia, and polyuria.

Specific Gravity

- Defined as weight of a volume of urine compared to equal volume of distilled water.
- Generally corresponds with the urine osmolality.
- However, if large molecules are present in the urine such as glucose and radiocontrast, then specific gravity will differ from the osmolality; in these cases, the use of the urine osmolality is preferred.

Glucose

- A positive glucose test result usually signifies one of two possibilities:
  - High concentration of glucose present in blood which results in the spilling of glucose into the urine
  - Normal concentration of glucose present in blood but filtered glucose is not reabsorbed because of impaired tubular function
- In the presence of normal renal function, glucosuria is typically not seen until plasma glucose exceeds 180 mg/dL.
- Glucosuria due to impaired tubular function is less common. It may be isolated or coexist with other abnormalities related to impaired tubular function such as aminoaciduria, hypophosphatemia, and hypouricemia. This constellation of findings is known as the renal Fanconi syndrome.
- Urine dipstick testing for glucose is not recommended for screening and monitoring of patients with diabetes mellitus.

Blood or Heme

- Positive dipstick test result for blood or heme should prompt consideration of hematuria, hemoglobinuria, or myoglobinuria.
- See hematuria *on page 171* for more information

Leukocyte Esterase

- A positive dipstick test result for leukocyte esterase signifies pyuria.
- The most common cause of pyuria is urinary tract infection.
- Therefore, positive dipstick test result for leukocyte esterase should prompt consideration of urinary tract infection, especially if the patient has signs and symptoms of urinary tract infection.
- There are noninfectious causes of pyuria; leukocyte esterase testing will be positive in these cases as well.
- Urine specimen that is positive for leukocyte esterase but negative for the presence of white blood cells on examination of the urine sediment suggests the possibility of cell lysis. White blood cell lysis is not uncommon in hypotonic or alkaline urine.

Nitrite

- A positive dipstick test result for nitrite suggests the presence of bacteria in the urine that can convert nitrates to nitrites.
- A positive test result is suggestive of urinary tract infection, especially in patients with signs and symptoms of urinary tract infection.

Bilirubin

- Bilirubin is not normally present in the urine.
- A positive urine dipstick for bilirubin signifies presence of conjugated hyperbilirubinemia.

Ketones

- Although small amounts of ketones are normally present in the urine, they are not normally detected by conventional dipstick testing.
- A positive dipstick test result for ketones indicates an excess of ketones.
- In diabetics, a positive urine dipstick test result for ketones should raise concern about the possibility of diabetic ketoacidosis.

URINE SEDIMENT

Microscopic examination of the urine sediment is done to identify cells, casts, crystals, and bacteria. It is not unusual to have small amounts of red blood cells (0-2 red blood cells/hpf) and white blood cells (0-4 white blood cells/hpf) present in normal urine.

Red Blood Cells

- It is normal to see a small amount of red blood cells in the urinary sediment
- The presence of >3 red blood cells per high powered field (spun urine sediment) is abnormal and satisfies the definition of hematuria
- In patients with extrarenal hematuria, the red blood cells are typically uniform and round.
- In patients with glomerular hematuria, dysmorphic red blood cells may be appreciated. The term "dysmorphic" refers to variability in red blood cell morphology (ie, blebs).

White Blood Cells

- The most common cause of pyuria is urinary tract infection.
- Noninfectious cause of pyuria should also be considered, especially when signs and symptoms of urinary tract infection or bacteriuria are absent.
- The presence of sterile pyuria should prompt consideration of genitourinary tuberculosis.
- Eosinophils and lymphocytes may also be present in the urine; Wright's stain is required to identify these types of white blood cells.
- Many feel that the presence of eosinophils is diagnostic of acute interstitial nephritis. Recent studies have suggested that eosinophiluria may be associated with other conditions.

Bacteria

- Normal urine is sterile.
- Presence of bacteria or bacteriuria signifies either infection or contamination.
- When accompanied by pyuria, bacteriuria very suggestive of urinary tract infection.
- The absence of pyuria in the patient with bacteriuria should prompt consideration of contamination or asymptomatic bacteriuria.

Crystals

- Occasionally, uric acid and calcium oxalate crystals may be found in normal urine.
- The presence of calcium oxalate crystals in patients presenting with acute renal failure and high anion gap metabolic acidosis should prompt consideration of ethylene glycol intoxication.
- The presence of cystine crystals is diagnostic of cystinuria.
- Magnesium ammonium phosphate crystals may be seen in the urine sediment of patients who have urinary tract infection due to urea-splitting organisms (ie, *Klebsiella, Proteus*).

Casts

- Red blood cell casts: Consider glomerular disease or vasculitis
- White blood cell casts: Consider acute pyelonephritis and tubulointerstitial disease
- Waxy or broad cast: Indicates advanced renal failure
- Hyaline casts: Not indicative of disease
- Epithelial cell cast: Increased numbers suggest acute tubular necrosis, acute glomerulonephritis, nephrotic syndrome, and pyelonephritis

GASTROENTEROLOGY

LIVER FUNCTION TESTS

The liver is a remarkable organ having a wide variety of functions. As such, it is not possible to evaluate liver function with a single laboratory test. Not uncommonly, the term "liver function tests" is used to refer to a battery of tests that often includes the following:

- Aspartate aminotransferase (AST)
- Alanine aminotransferase (ALT)
- Alkaline phosphatase
- Gamma-glutamyltransferase (GGT)
- 5′ nucleotidase
- Bilirubin
- Albumin
- Prothrombin time (PT)

These tests will be discussed in more detail in the pages that follow.

ASPARTATE AMINOTRANSFERASE (AST) / ALANINE AMINOTRANSFERASE (ALT)

AST and ALT, previously known as serum glutamic oxaloacetic transaminase (SGOT) and serum glutamic pyruvic transaminase (SGPT), respectively, are enzymes found in the liver cell. With hepatocellular damage or necrosis, AST and ALT levels may rise.

Sensitivity of AST and ALT in the Detection of Liver Disease

Liver disease is not excluded in the patient with normal AST and ALT levels. Examples of this include the following:

- Cirrhosis (in the absence of ongoing liver cell injury)
- Chronic hepatitis C (some patients have persistently normal AST and ALT levels)
- Uremia (upper limit of normal in patients on hemodialysis is about 50% of that appreciated in healthy individuals)

Specificity of AST and ALT in the Detection of Liver Disease

- AST and ALT are not entirely specific for the liver
- Both are found in many other organs
- Of the two, ALT elevation is more specific for liver disease

Conditions Associated With Marked Transaminase Elevation (>1000 units/L)

- Acute viral hepatitis
- Drugs / toxins
- Ischemic hepatitis
- Acute biliary obstruction
- Autoimmune hepatitis

Conditions Associated With Mild to Moderate Transaminase Elevation

- Differential diagnosis of mild to moderate transaminase elevation is more extensive than that for marked transaminase elevation.
- Of note, transaminase levels seldom climb to >400 units/L in alcoholic liver disease (suspect other causes of liver disease if alcoholic patient presents with this degree of transaminase elevation).

AST:ALT Ratio >1

- Major consideration is alcoholic liver disease.
- Ratio >2 is even more suggestive of alcoholic liver disease.
- AST:ALT ratio >1 is not pathognomonic for alcoholic liver disease as other types of liver disease may also present with this type of ratio.
- Alcoholic liver disease may also present with ratio <1.
- AST:ALT ratio >1 also seen in cirrhosis, irrespective of the etiology.

AST:ALT Ratio <1

- ALT:AST ratio >1 in most types of liver disease.
- Exceptions are alcoholic liver disease, Reye's syndrome, and cirrhosis, irrespective of the etiology.

Degree of Transaminase Elevation and Prognosis

- There is no correlation between the degree of transaminase elevation and extent of hepatocellular necrosis.
- Height of transaminase elevation has no bearing on patient's prognosis.

APPROACH TO THE ASYMPTOMATIC PATIENT WITH MILD TRANSAMINASE ELEVATION

Major Hepatic Causes of Mild Transaminase Elevation

- Alcoholic liver disease
- Chronic hepatitis B
- Chronic hepatitis C
- Autoimmune hepatitis
- Fatty liver (hepatic steatosis)
- Nonalcoholic steatohepatitis
- Cirrhosis
- Hemochromatosis
- Wilson's disease
- α1-antitrypsin deficiency
- Drug-induced liver disease
- Congestive hepatopathy
- Acute viral hepatitis (AE, EBV, CMV)
- Celiac disease

APPROACH TO THE ASYMPTOMATIC PATIENT WITH MILDLY ELEVATED TRANSAMINASE LEVELS

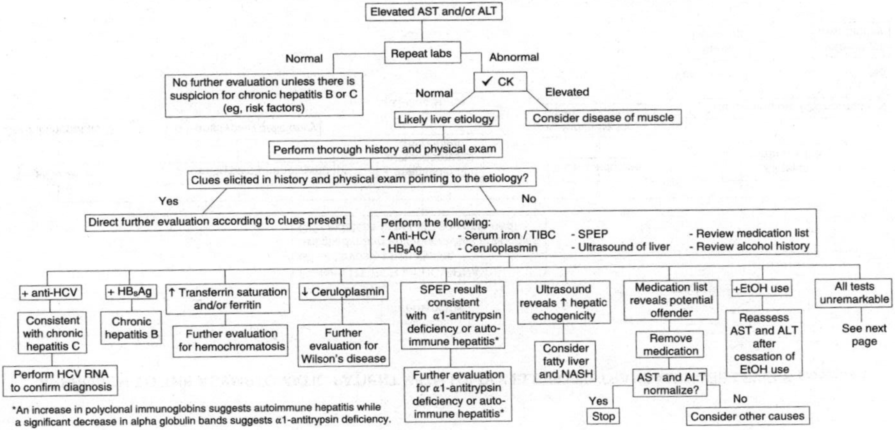
Elevated AST and/or ALT
Repeat labs
Normal
Abnormal
No further evaluation unless there is suspicion for chronic hepatitis B or C (eg, risk factors)
✓ CK
Normal
Elevated
Likely liver etiology
Consider disease of muscle
Perform thorough history and physical exam
Clues elicited in history and physical exam pointing to the etiology?
Yes
No
Direct further evaluation according to clues present
Perform the following:
- Anti-HCV
- HB_sAg
- Serum iron / TIBC
- Ceruloplasmin
- SPEP
- Ultrasound of liver
- Review medication list
- Review alcohol history
+ anti-HCV
Consistent with chronic hepatitis C
Perform HCV RNA to confirm diagnosis
+ HB_sAg
Chronic hepatitis B
↑ Transferrin saturation and/or ferritin
Further evaluation for hemochromatosis
↓ Ceruloplasmin
Further evaluation for Wilson's disease
SPEP results consistent with α1-antitrypsin deficiency or auto-immune hepatitis*
Further evaluation for α1-antitrypsin deficiency or auto-immune hepatitis*
Ultrasound reveals ↑ hepatic echogenicity
Consider fatty liver and NASH
Medication list reveals potential offender
Remove medication
AST and ALT normalize?
Yes
Stop
No
Consider other causes
+EtOH use
Reassess AST and ALT after cessation of EtOH use
All tests unremarkable

See next page

*An increase in polyclonal immunoglobins suggests autoimmune hepatitis while a significant decrease in alpha globulin bands suggests α1-antitrypsin deficiency.

APPROACH TO THE ASYMPTOMATIC PATIENT WITH MILDLY ELEVATED TRANSAMINASE LEVELS *(continued)*

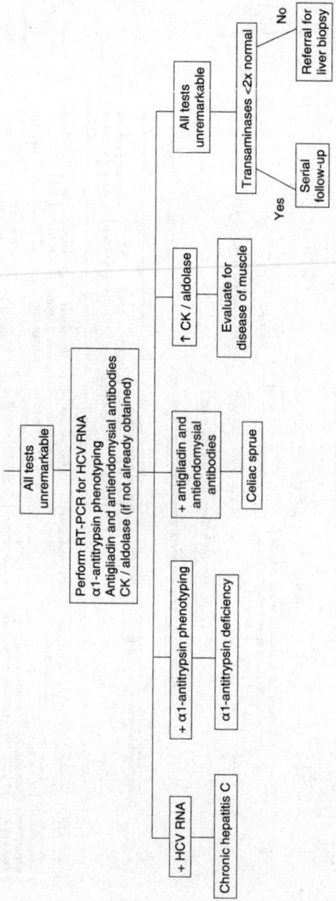

All tests unremarkable
Perform RT-PCR for HCV RNA
α1-antitrypsin phenotyping
Antigliadin and antiendomysial antibodies
CK / aldolase (if not already obtained)
+ HCV RNA
Chronic hepatitis C
+ α1-antitrypsin phenotyping
α1-antitrypsin deficiency
+ antigliadin and antiendomysial antibodies
Celiac sprue
↑ CK / aldolase
Evaluate for disease of muscle
All tests unremarkable
Transaminases <2x normal
Yes
Serial follow-up
No
Referral for liver biopsy

ALBUMIN

Albumin is synthesized exclusively by the liver. In the blood, albumin exerts a significant osmotic effect and is integral in the transport of both endogenous and exogenous substances.

Causes of Elevated Serum Albumin Level

- Dehydration
- Prolonged tourniquet use during collection
- Specimen evaporation

Causes of Hypoalbuminemia

- Malnutrition
- Malabsorption
- Malignancy
- Inflammation (acute or chronic)
- Increased loss
  - Nephrotic syndrome
  - Protein-losing enteropathy
  - Burns
  - Exudative skin disease
- Intravenous fluids
- Rapid hydration
- Overhydration
- Cirrhosis
- Chronic liver disease
- Pregnancy

Sensitivity and Specificity of Serum Albumin Level in the Diagnosis of Liver Disease

- Liver is the only source of albumin production.
- Half-life of albumin is 3 weeks.
- Because of the long half-life, serum albumin levels are a much better gauge of synthetic function in chronic liver disease.
- In cases of acute hepatic necrosis, the serum albumin level may not accurately reflect the true derangement in liver function.

- Even in patients with chronic liver disease and cirrhosis, serum albumin levels may be normal. This is because the liver can increase albumin synthesis as much as twofold in response to any process that impairs its synthetic function.
- There are many nonhepatic conditions associated with hypoalbuminemia (see list above)

PROTHROMBIN TIME (PT)

Prothrombin time is a measure of the function of the extrinsic pathway. The factors integral to the determination of the PT are made in the liver.

Sensitivity of the PT in the Detection of Liver Disease

- PT is a marker of the liver's synthetic function.
- Despite this, it will remain normal until at least 80% of the liver's synthetic ability is compromised.
- For this reason, PT is normal in many patients with chronic liver disease and cirrhosis.
- When compared to albumin, PT is more useful gauge of synthetic function in acute liver disease. This is because the coagulation factors integral to PT determination have shorter half-lives (hours) than albumin (3 weeks).

Specificity of the PT in the Detection of Liver Disease

- Elevated PT is not specific for liver disease since there are other causes.
- Causes of an isolated elevation of PT include the following:
  - Vitamin K deficiency
  - Warfarin
  - Liver disease
  - Factor VII deficiency (inherited or acquired)
  - False-positive test result (inadequate tube filling, high hematocrit)
- It is usually not difficult to determine the cause of the isolated elevation of PT:
  - Warfarin use is typically apparent
  - Factor VII deficiency is quite rare
  - If false-positive test result is not likely, two major considerations are vitamin K deficiency and liver disease
  - To differentiate between vitamin K deficiency and liver disease, give parenteral vitamin K (10 mg subcutaneously). A decrease in PT of at least 30% within 24 hours of administration consistent with vitamin K deficiency.
  - It is important to realize that both vitamin K deficiency and liver disease may coexist

ALKALINE PHOSPHATASE

Alkaline phosphatase is an enzyme that catalyzes the hydrolysis of phosphate esters at an alkaline pH. Alkaline phosphatase is found in many organs, including the liver and biliary tree, bone, placenta, intestine, and kidney. Increases in alkaline phosphatase may be seen in tissues that are active in metabolism. Adolescence and pregnancy are, therefore, states when alkaline phosphatase may be elevated due to bone and placental growth, respectively. Clinically, elevations in alkaline phosphatase are usually of hepatobiliary or bone origin.

Causes of an Elevated Alkaline Phosphatase

- Cholestasis
  - Intrahepatic
    - Medication-induced
    - Primary biliary cirrhosis
    - Benign recurrent intrahepatic cholestasis
    - Intrahepatic cholestasis of pregnancy
    - Total parenteral nutrition
    - Cholestasis of sepsis
    - Alcoholic hepatitis
    - Postoperative cholestasis
    - Systemic infection
    - Viral hepatitis
  - Extrahepatic
    - Stones
    - Biliary stricture
    - Malignancy
      - Pancreatic
      - Ampullary
      - Duodenal
      - Cholangiocarcinoma
      - Lymphoma
      - Metastases to portal lymph nodes
    - Pancreatitis / pancreatic pseudocyst
    - Primary sclerosing cholangitis
    - Biliary malformation
    - AIDS cholangiopathy

- Infiltrative disease of the liver
  - Granulomatous disease (tuberculosis, sarcoidosis, etc)
  - Amyloidosis
  - Leukemia
  - Lymphoma

- Mass lesions of the liver
  - Malignancy (hepatoma, metastatic cancer)
  - Cyst
  - Abscess
- Parenchymal disease of the liver
  - Viral hepatitis (acute or chronic)
  - Alcoholic liver disease
  - Hereditary liver disease (hemochromatosis, Wilson's disease, α1-antitrypsin deficiency)
  - Cirrhosis
  - Congestive hepatopathy
  - Autoimmune hepatitis
  - Medication-induced
  - Ischemic hepatitis
  - Hepatic steatosis
- Bone disease
  - Fractures
  - Paget's disease
  - Rickets
  - Osteomalacia
  - Osteitis fibrosa cystica
  - Osteoblastic bone tumors (osteogenic sarcoma, metastatic tumors)
  - Bone growth (childhood and adolescence)
- Miscellaneous
  - Malignancy (renal cell carcinoma, lymphoma)
  - Hyperthyroidism
  - Acromegaly
  - Myelofibrosis
  - Mastocytosis
  - Hypervitaminosis D
  - Pulmonary infarct
  - Renal infarction
  - AIDS
  - *C. difficile* infection in AIDS patients

APPROACH TO THE PATIENT WITH AN ALKALINE PHOSPHATASE ELEVATION OUT OF PROPORTION TO THE TRANSAMINASE ELEVATION

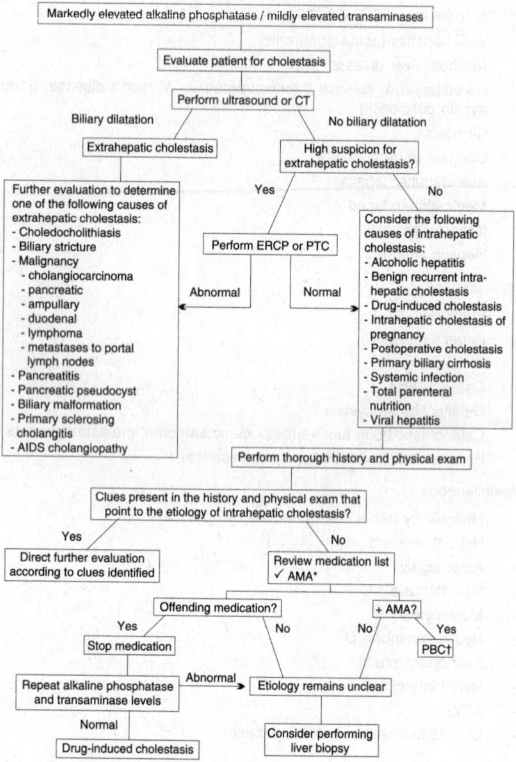
Markedly elevated alkaline phosphatase / mildly elevated transaminases
Evaluate patient for cholestasis
Perform ultrasound or CT
Biliary dilatation
No biliary dilatation
Extrahepatic cholestasis
High suspicion for extrahepatic cholestasis?
Yes
No
Further evaluation to determine one of the following causes of extrahepatic cholestasis:
- Choledocholithiasis
- Biliary stricture
- Malignancy
- cholangiocarcinoma
- pancreatic
- ampullary
- duodenal
- lymphoma
- metastases to portal lymph nodes
- Pancreatitis
- Pancreatic pseudocyst
- Biliary malformation
- Primary sclerosing cholangitis
- AIDS cholangiopathy
Perform ERCP or PTC
Abnormal
Normal
Consider the following causes of intrahepatic cholestasis:
- Alcoholic hepatitis
- Benign recurrent intra-hepatic cholestasis
- Drug-induced cholestasis
- Intrahepatic cholestasis of pregnancy
- Postoperative cholestasis
- Primary biliary cirrhosis
- Systemic infection
- Total parenteral nutrition
- Viral hepatitis
Perform thorough history and physical exam
Clues present in the history and physical exam that point to the etiology of intrahepatic cholestasis?
Yes
No
Direct further evaluation according to clues identified
Review medication list
✓ AMA*
Offending medication?
+ AMA?
Yes
No
No
Yes
Stop medication
PBC†
Repeat alkaline phosphatase and transaminase levels
Abnormal
Etiology remains unclear
Normal
Drug-induced cholestasis
Consider performing liver biopsy

* AMA = antimitochrondrial antibody
† PBC = primary biliary cirrhosis

APPROACH TO THE PATIENT WITH ISOLATED ELEVATION OF ALKALINE PHOSPHATASE

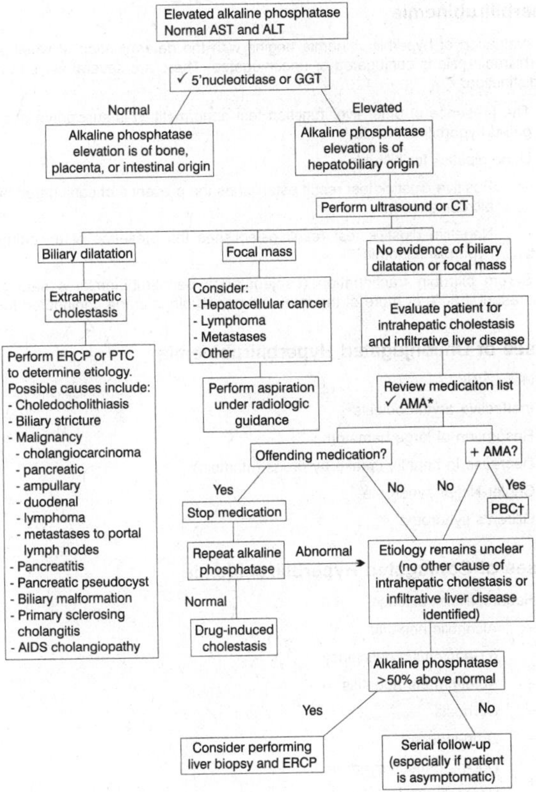
Elevated alkaline phosphatase
Normal AST and ALT
✓ 5'nucleotidase or GGT
Normal
Elevated
Alkaline phosphatase elevation is of bone, placenta, or intestinal origin
Alkaline phosphatase elevation is of hepatobiliary origin
Perform ultrasound or CT
Biliary dilatation
Focal mass
No evidence of biliary dilatation or focal mass
Extrahepatic cholestasis
Consider:
- Hepatocellular cancer
- Lymphoma
- Metastases
- Other
Evaluate patient for intrahepatic cholestasis and infiltrative liver disease
Perform ERCP or PTC to determine etiology.
Possible causes include:
- Choledocholithiasis
- Biliary stricture
- Malignancy
- cholangiocarcinoma
- pancreatic
- ampullary
- duodenal
- lymphoma
- metastases to portal lymph nodes
- Pancreatitis
- Pancreatic pseudocyst
- Biliary malformation
- Primary sclerosing cholangitis
- AIDS cholangiopathy
Perform aspiration under radiologic guidance
Review medicaiton list
✓ AMA*
Offending medication?
+ AMA?
Yes
No
No
Yes
PBC†
Stop medication
Repeat alkaline phosphatase
Abnormal
Etiology remains unclear (no other cause of intrahepatic cholestasis or infiltrative liver disease identified)
Normal
Drug-induced cholestasis
Alkaline phosphatase >50% above normal
Yes
No
Consider performing liver biopsy and ERCP
Serial follow-up (especially if patient is asymptomatic)

* AMA = antimitochondrial antibody
† PBC = primary biliary cirrhosis

BILIRUBIN

Differentiating Conjugated From Unconjugated Hyperbilirubinemia

The evaluation of hyperbilirubinemia begins with the determination of whether the hyperbilirubinemia is conjugated or unconjugated. There are several ways to make this distinction:

- The presence of other liver function test abnormalities is supportive of conjugated hyperbilirubinemia
- Urine dipstick for bilirubin
  - Positive dipstick test result establishes the presence of conjugated hyperbilirubinemia
  - Negative dipstick test result establishes the presence of unconjugated hyperbilirubinemia
- Serum bilirubin fractionation (conjugated hyperbilirubinemia is said to be present if 30% or more of the total serum bilirubin is in the conjugated form)

Causes of Unconjugated Hyperbilirubinemia

- Hemolysis
- Ineffective erythropoiesis
- Resorption of large hematoma
- Decrease in hepatic uptake by drugs (rifampin)
- Crigler-Najjar syndrome
- Gilbert's syndrome

Causes of Conjugated Hyperbilirubinemia

- Hepatocellular disease
  - Alcoholic hepatitis
  - α1-antitrypsin deficiency
  - Autoimmune hepatitis
  - Cirrhosis
  - Drug-induced
  - Dubin-Johnson syndrome
  - Hemochromatosis
  - Hepatotoxins
  - Hepatic vein thrombosis

- Ischemia
- Rotor's syndrome
- Viral hepatitis
- Wilson's disease

- Cholestasis
  - Extrahepatic
    - AIDS cholangiopathy
    - Biliary malformation
    - Choledocholithiasis
    - Malignancy
      - Ampullary
      - Cholangiocarcinoma
      - Duodenal
      - Lymphoma
      - Metastases to portal lymph nodes
      - Pancreatic
    - Pancreatic pseudocyst
    - Pancreatitis
    - Primary sclerosing cholangitis
  - Intrahepatic
    - Alcoholic hepatitis
    - Benign recurrent intrahepatic cholestasis
    - Cholestasis of pregnancy
    - Drug-induced
    - Postoperative hyperbilirubinemia
    - Primary biliary cirrhosis
    - Systemic infection
    - Total parenteral nutrition
    - Viral hepatitis

APPROACH TO THE PATIENT WITH HYPERBILIRUBINEMIA

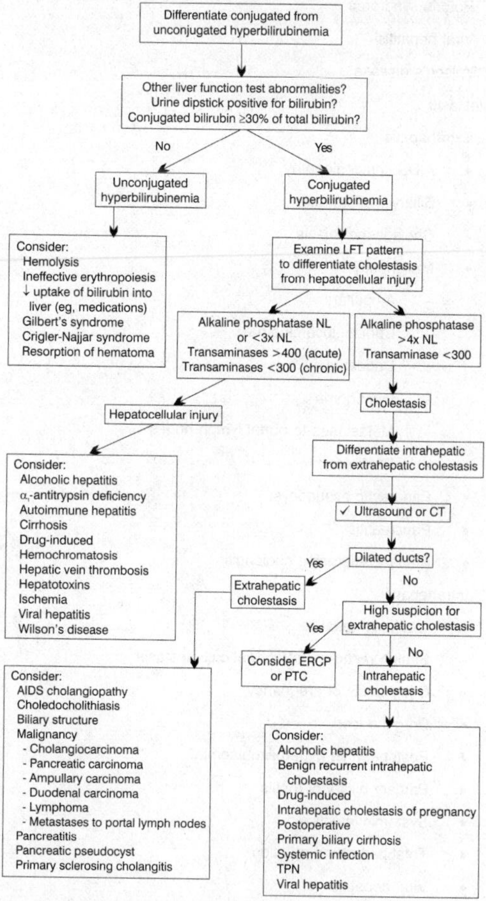
Differentiate conjugated from unconjugated hyperbilirubinemia
Other liver function test abnormalities? Urine dipstick positive for bilirubin? Conjugated bilirubin ≥30% of total bilirubin?
No
Yes
Unconjugated hyperbilirubinemia
Conjugated hyperbilirubinemia
Consider: Hemolysis Ineffective erythropoiesis ↓ uptake of bilirubin into liver (eg, medications) Gilbert's syndrome Crigler-Najjar syndrome Resorption of hematoma
Examine LFT pattern to differentiate cholestasis from hepatocellular injury
Alkaline phosphatase NL or <3x NL Transaminases >400 (acute) Transaminases <300 (chronic)
Alkaline phosphatase >4x NL Transaminase <300
Hepatocellular injury
Cholestasis
Consider: Alcoholic hepatitis α_1-antitrypsin deficiency Autoimmune hepatitis Cirrhosis Drug-induced Hemochromatosis Hepatic vein thrombosis Hepatotoxins Ischemia Viral hepatitis Wilson's disease
Differentiate intrahepatic from extrahepatic cholestasis
✓ Ultrasound or CT
Dilated ducts?
Yes
Extrahepatic cholestasis
No
High suspicion for extrahepatic cholestasis
Yes
No
Consider ERCP or PTC
Intrahepatic cholestasis
Consider: AIDS cholangiopathy Choledocholithiasis Biliary structure Malignancy - Cholangiocarcinoma - Pancreatic carcinoma - Ampullary carcinoma - Duodenal carcinoma - Lymphoma - Metastases to portal lymph nodes Pancreatitis Pancreatic pseudocyst Primary sclerosing cholangitis
Consider: Alcoholic hepatitis Benign recurrent intrahepatic cholestasis Drug-induced Intrahepatic cholestasis of pregnancy Postoperative Primary biliary cirrhosis Systemic infection TPN Viral hepatitis

5′ NUCLEOTIDASE

An isolated increase in the alkaline phosphatase level is the only indication for the measurement of a 5′ nucleotidase level. In these patients, the elevated alkaline phosphatase level may be of hepatobiliary or bone origin. To differentiate between these two sources of alkaline phosphatase elevation, a 5′ nucleotidase level may be obtained. If the 5′ nucleotidase level is elevated, then some type of hepatobiliary disease is the etiology of the alkaline phosphatase elevation. If the 5′ nucleotidase level is normal, then the clinician should focus on bone diseases that are associated with alkaline phosphatase elevation.

GAMMA GLUTAMYL TRANSFERASE (GGT)

- GGT is elevated in many types of hepatic disease; therefore, its use in differentiating among different types of liver disease is limited.
- GGT does have a role in the evaluation of patients presenting with isolated alkaline phosphatase elevation. In these patients, the alkaline phosphatase elevation may be of hepatobiliary or bone origin. If the GGT level is elevated, then the alkaline phosphatase elevation is of hepatobiliary origin. If the GGT level is normal, then the clinician should focus on bone diseases that present with an elevated alkaline phosphatase level.
- GGT is not specific for liver disease because an elevated level may reflect disease in other organs such as the kidney, pancreas, and intestines.
- GGT is induced by a number of drugs. Drug-induced GGT elevation is seen with the use of carbamazepine, cimetidine, furosemide, heparin, isotretinoin, methotrexate, oral contraceptives, phenobarbital, phenytoin, and valproic acid.
- There is a direct relationship between alcohol intake and GGT. GGT levels may remain increased for weeks after cessation of chronic alcohol intake.

AMMONIA

The final product of amino acid and nucleic acid metabolism is ammonia. The liver is the only organ that detoxifies ammonia by converting it into urea.

Sensitivity of Ammonia Level in the Detection of Hepatic Encephalopathy

- Although ammonia levels have been used to provide support for the diagnosis of hepatic encephalopathy, they are not recommended for the diagnosis because some patients have normal ammonia levels.
- A normal ammonia level does not exclude the diagnosis of hepatic encephalopathy.

Specificity of Ammonia Level in the Detection of Hepatic Encephalopathy

The presence of an elevated ammonia level does not establish the diagnosis of hepatic encephalopathy. There are many other causes of an elevated ammonia level:

- Hepatocellular dysfunction
- Excessive bleeding
- Excessive dietary protein
- Constipation
- Renal insufficiency
- Alkalosis
- Portosystemic venous shunt
- Hypokalemia
- Acute leukemia
- Blood transfusion
- Bone marrow transplantation
- Medications (valproic acid, glycine)
- Hemodialysis
- Ureterosigmoidostomy
- Asparaginase therapy

ALPHA-FETOPROTEIN (AFP)

- AFP levels are increased in >90% of patients with hepatocellular cancer (50% to 80% have elevated AFP levels at the time of presentation).
- AFP elevation is not entirely specific for hepatocellular cancer.
- AFP may also be elevated in patients with acute liver disease, chronic liver disease, cirrhosis, and hepatic metastases.
- An AFP level >500 ng/mL (especially in the presence of a liver mass) is strongly suggestive of hepatocellular cancer.
- In patients with chronic liver disease / cirrhosis, serial measurement of AFP levels are useful in hepatocellular cancer screening.
- AFP levels are also useful in monitoring the response to therapy of hepatocellular cancer.

ACUTE VIRAL HEPATITIS

Laboratory Features of Acute Viral Hepatitis

- Increased transaminases
  - Levels peak near the onset of jaundice
  - Gradual fall in levels occur after peaking
  - Once levels are noted to consistently decrease, no need to measure levels until signs and symptoms of acute viral hepatitis have resolved
- Increased bilirubin
  - Peaking of serum bilirubin levels typically occur 1 week after transaminase levels peak
  - Only 4% have peak levels >20 mg/dL
- Increased alkaline phosphatase
  - Seldom does the level exceed three times the upper limit of normal
- PT / PTT usually normal
  - Increased PT and PTT uncommon
  - Elevated PT and PTT should prompt consideration of severe, subfulminant, or fulminant disease
- Mild anemia
- Decreased WBC count (WBC count >12,000 cells mm^3 rare)
- Atypical lymphocytes
- Relative lymphocytosis
- Decreased platelet count
- Increased ferritin
- Increased serum iron
- Increased ESR
- Rare complications
  - Pure red cell aplasia
  - Aplastic anemia
  - Membranous glomerulonephritis
  - DIC
  - Agranulocytosis
  - Hemolytic anemia

Essential Viral Serology in Acute Viral Hepatitis

- Hepatitis A
  - Obtain IgM anti-HAV
  - Occasionally IgM anti-HAV is undetectable at the time of testing. In these patients, it is worthwhile to repeat testing in 1-2 weeks.
- Hepatitis B
  - Obtain HB_sAg and IgM anti-HB_c
  - Other hepatitis B viral markers and antibodies are not useful in the diagnosis of acute hepatitis B viral infection
- Hepatitis C
  - Obtain anti-HCV
  - There are several limitations of anti-HCV testing in the diagnosis of acute hepatitis C viral infection. When second generation enzyme immunoassays (EIA-II) tests are used, 80% to 90% of patients with acute hepatitis C will be diagnosed by the presence of detectable anti-HCV. To detect the remaining patients, the clinician may elect to repeat the anti-HCV test in order to demonstrate conversion from negative to positive. Alternatively, the clinician may wish to obtain HCV RNA. Positive HCV RNA also supports the diagnosis of acute hepatitis C viral infection.

Testing for hepatitis D and E should be individualized. For example, testing for acute hepatitis D viral infection should be obtained in patients with positive HB_sAg who present with severe acute hepatitis or a biphasic pattern of illness. Acute hepatitis E viral infection should be a consideration mainly in patients who report a history of recent travel or in new immigrants with acute hepatic injury.

HEPATITIS A

Liver Function Tests in Acute Hepatitis A Viral Infection

Liver function test abnormalities do not allow the clinician to distinguish acute hepatitis A viral infection from other causes of viral hepatitis. Liver function test abnormalities as well as other laboratory test findings in acute viral hepatitis are discussed in more detail *on page 213.*

Establishing the Diagnosis of Acute Hepatitis A Viral Infection

- Diagnosis is based on the presence of IgM anti-HAV antibody.
- IgM anti-HAV antibody appears 1-2 weeks after exposure.
- Presence of IgM anti-HAV antibody is indicative of recent or current hepatitis A viral infection (within the past 6 months).
- On occasion, the test is negative at the time of presentation. In these patients, a repeat test done 1-2 weeks later usually reveals the presence of the antibody.
- IgM anti-HAV antibody typically disappears by 6 months.
- Persistence of IgM anti-HAV has been described for up to 1 year.
- IgG anti-HAV antibody is detectable 5-6 weeks after exposure.
- IgG anti-HAV antibody remains positive indefinitely.

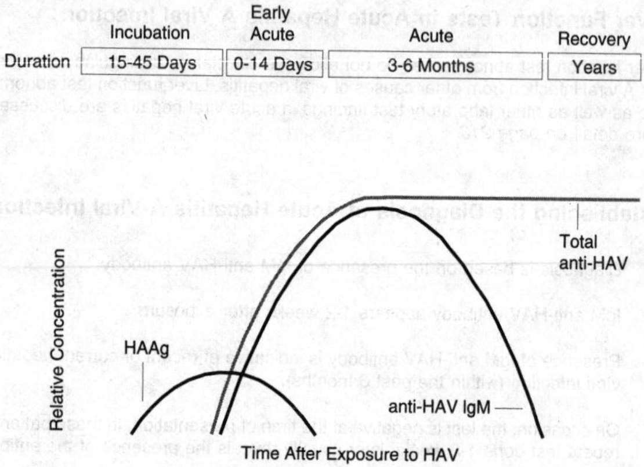
Early
Incubation
Acute
Acute
Recovery
Duration
15-45 Days
0-14 Days
3-6 Months
Years
Total
anti-HAV
Relative Concentration
HAAg
anti-HAV IgM
Time After Exposure to HAV

Reprinted from Abbott Diagnostics

ACUTE HEPATITIS B VIRAL INFECTION

Liver Function Test Abnormalities in Acute Hepatitis B Viral Infection

Liver function test abnormalities do not allow the clinician to distinguish acute hepatitis B viral infection from other causes of viral hepatitis. Liver function test abnormalities as well as other laboratory test findings in acute viral hepatitis are discussed in more detail *on page 213.*

Establishing the Diagnosis of Acute Hepatitis B Viral Infection

- Tests that should be ordered to confirm the diagnosis of acute hepatitis B viral infection include HB_sAg and IgM anti-HB_c.
- Most patients will have positive HB_sAg.
- Ten percent, however, will present at a time in their illness when HB_sAg is negative. A positive IgM anti-HB_c will establish the diagnosis in these patients. These patients are said to be in the window period (period of time between the disappearance of HB_sAg and appearance of anti-HB_s).
- No other serologic markers of hepatitis B are needed to establish the diagnosis of acute hepatitis B viral infection.

HEPATITIS B PROFILE

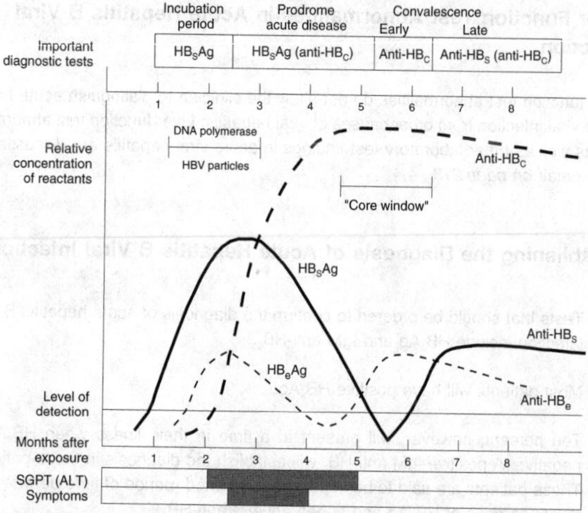
Incubation period
Prodrome acute disease
Convalescence
Early
Late
Important diagnostic tests
HBsAg
HBsAg (anti-HBc)
Anti-HBc
Anti-HBs (anti-HBc)
1
2
3
4
5
6
7
8
DNA polymerase
HBV particles
Relative concentration of reactants
Anti-HBc
"Core window"
HBsAg
Anti-HBs
HBeAg
Anti-HBe
Level of detection
Months after exposure
SGPT (ALT)
Symptoms

Serologic and clinical patterns observed during acute hepatitis B viral infection. From Hollinger FB and Dreesman GR, *Manual of Clinical Immunology*, 2nd ed, Rose NR and Friedman H, eds, Washington, DC: American Society for Microbiology, 1980, with permission.

CHRONIC HEPATITIS B VIRAL INFECTION

When HB_sAg persists for more than 6 months, a diagnosis of chronic hepatitis B has been established. Overall, recovery from acute hepatitis B occurs in >95% of patients. In the remaining 5% of patients, hepatitis B persists either as chronic (replicative) hepatitis or as an asymptomatic chronic (nonreplicative) carrier state.

Liver Function Tests in Chronic Hepatitis B Viral Infection

- Transaminase levels may be completely normal in chronic hepatitis B.
- Most patients, however, have mild to moderate transaminase elevation.
- Occasionally, transaminase levels climb markedly with exacerbations.
- The presence of leukopenia, thrombocytopenia, hypoalbuminemia, or increased PT suggests progression of liver disease to cirrhosis.

Establishing the Diagnosis of Chronic Hepatitis B Viral Infection

- Diagnosis is established when persistence of HB_sAg in the serum for over 6 months is demonstrated.
- Once diagnosis is established, further serologic testing is recommended to determine if patient has replicative or nonreplicative infection.
- Serologic testing consistent with replicative infection includes the following:
  - + HBV DNA
  - + HB_eAg
  - + HB_sAg
  - - Anti-HB_s
  - - Anti-HB_e
  - + Anti-HB_c
- Serologic testing consistent with nonreplicative infection includes the following:
  - - HBV DNA
  - - HB_eAg
  - + HB_sAg
  - - Anti-HB_s
  - + Anti-HB_e
  - + Anti-HB_c
- Many patients cycle back and forth between the replicative and nonreplicative state. With transformation of the replicative state into the nonreplicative state, HB_eAg is lost and anti-HB_e is detected in the serum.

Hepatitis B Chronic (Replicative) State

No Seroconversion

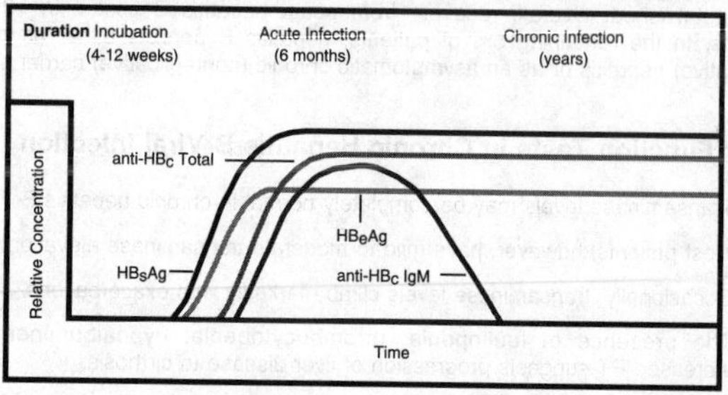
Duration Incubation
(4-12 weeks)
Acute Infection
(6 months)
Chronic Infection
(years)
Relative Concentration
anti-HBc Total
HBeAg
HBsAg
anti-HBc IgM
Time

Hepatitis B Chronic (Nonreplicative) Carrier

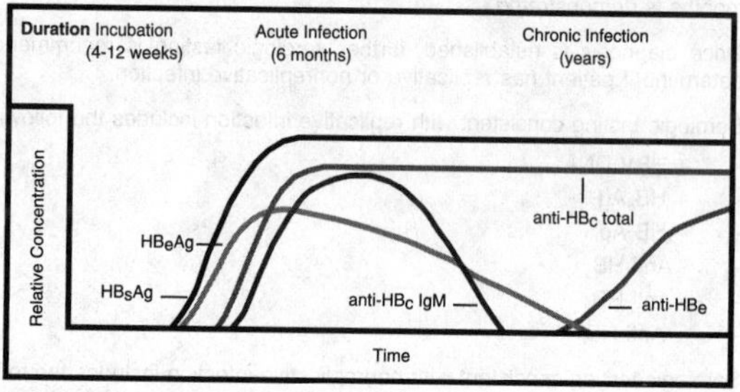
Duration Incubation
(4-12 weeks)
Acute Infection
(6 months)
Chronic Infection
(years)
Relative Concentration
anti-HBc total
HBeAg
HBsAg
anti-HBc IgM
anti-HBe
Time

ACUTE HEPATITIS C VIRAL INFECTION

Liver Function Test Abnormalities in Acute Hepatitis C Viral Infection

Liver function test abnormalities do not allow the clinician to distinguish acute hepatitis C viral infection from other causes of viral hepatitis. Liver function test abnormalities as well as other laboratory test findings in acute viral hepatitis are discussed in more detail *on page 213.*

Establishing the Diagnosis of Acute Hepatitis C Viral Infection

- The diagnosis of acute hepatitis C viral infection can be confirmed by testing for anti-HCV or HCV RNA.
- Because anti-HCV is readily available, easily performed, and relatively inexpensive, it is the preferred test for the diagnosis of acute hepatitis C viral infection.
- The percentage of patients who have detectable anti-HCV is related to the time since exposure:
  - 80% have detectable anti-HCV within 15 weeks of exposure
  - >90% have detectable anti-HCV within 5 months of exposure
  - >97% have detectable anti-HCV within 6 months of exposure
- Because anti-HCV may be undetectable for weeks or months after acquisition of the infection, the clinician may choose to repeat anti-HCV testing after a sufficient period of time if acute hepatitis C viral infection is suspected and the initial anti-HCV test is negative. Alternatively, the clinician can test for HCV RNA which is usually detectable within days of the acquisition of the virus.

Resolution of Acute Hepatitis C Viral Infection

- Only 15% to 20% of patients who acquire hepatitis C will recover from their illness.
- The majority will go on to develop chronic hepatitis C viral infection.

Figure 1.
Time Course of Serologic Markers in Acute Hepatitis C Infection

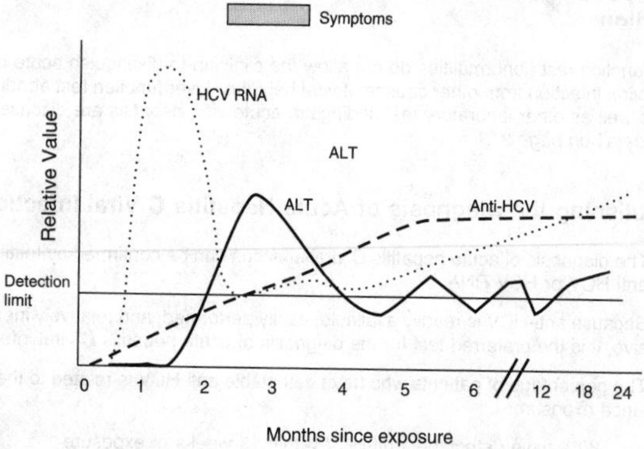

Symptoms
HCV RNA
ALT
ALT
Anti-HCV
Relative Value
Detection limit
0
1
2
3
4
5
6
12
18
24
Months since exposure

Adapted from Dufour DR, Lott JA, Nolte FS, et al, "Diagnosis and Monitoring of Hepatic Injury. I. Performance Characteristics of Laboratory Tests," *Clin Chem*, 2000, 46(12):2041.

CHRONIC HEPATITIS C VIRAL INFECTION

Eighty percent to 85% of patients who acquire hepatitis C go on to develop chronic hepatitis C.

Liver Function Tests in Chronic Hepatitis C Viral Infection

- Many patients with chronic hepatitis C viral infection have mild to moderate transaminase elevation.
- Some present with normal AST and ALT levels; therefore, normal transaminase levels do not exclude the diagnosis.
- Chronic hepatitis C viral infection is a well known cause of fluctuations in AST and ALT levels; that is transaminase levels fluctuate between normal and abnormal.

Establishing the Diagnosis of Chronic Hepatitis C Viral Infection

- A positive anti-HCV cannot be used to establish the diagnosis of chronic hepatitis C viral infection because the antibody is detectable in not only chronic hepatitis C patients but also in patients who have recovered from hepatitis C.
- To distinguish the 15% to 20% who have recovered from the 80% to 85% who have chronic hepatitis C viral infection, testing for HCV RNA must be performed.
  - Positive test result confirms the diagnosis of chronic hepatitis C viral infection
  - Negative test result should prompt the clinician to repeat the test as intermittent viremia is not uncommon

AMYLASE

Causes of Increased Serum Amylase

- Pancreatic disease
  - Pancreatitis
  - Pseudocyst
  - Abscess
  - Carcinoma
  - Ductal obstruction
  - Trauma (including surgery and ERCP)
  - Early cystic fibrosis
- Salivary disease
  - Infection (mumps)
  - Trauma (including surgery)
  - Radiation
  - Ductal obstruction
  - Tumor
- Gastrointestinal disease
  - Perforated / penetrating peptic ulcer
  - Mesenteric ischemia / infarction
  - Intestinal obstruction
  - Gut perforation (stomach, small intestine, large intestine)
  - Acute appendicitis
  - Acute cholecystitis
  - Common bile duct obstruction
  - Esophageal perforation
  - Hepatitis
  - Cirrhosis
  - Abdominal trauma with hematoma formation
  - Afferent loop obstruction
- Gynecologic disease
  - Ruptured ectopic pregnancy
  - Pelvic inflammatory disease
  - Ovarian cysts
  - Fallopian cysts

- Malignancy
  - Solid tumors (ovary, lung, esophagus, prostate, breast, thymus)
  - Multiple myeloma
  - Pheochromocytoma
- Miscellaneous
  - Renal failure
  - Diabetic ketoacidosis
  - Anorexia nervosa
  - Macroamylasemia
  - Cerebral trauma
  - Burns
  - Postoperative
  - Pregnancy
  - Ruptured aortic aneurysm or dissection
  - Postictical
  - Alcohol use
- Medications
  - Sphincter of Oddi spasm
    - Cholinergics
    - Bethanechol
    - Codeine
    - Morphine
    - Fentanyl
    - Meperidine
    - Pentazocine
    - Other narcotics
  - Parotitis
    - Phenylbutazone (causes parotitis)
    - Potassium iodide (causes parotitis)
    - Procyclidine
  - Drugs causing pancreatitis

LIPASE

Causes of Serum Lipase Elevation

- Pancreatic disease
  - Acute pancreatitis
  - Chronic pancreatitis
  - Post-ERCP / trauma
  - Calculus
  - Carcinoma
  - Abscess
  - Pseudocyst
- Gastrointestinal / hepatobiliary disease
  - Intestinal ischemia / infarction
  - Intestinal obstruction
  - Acute appendicitis
  - Acute cholecystitis
  - Common bile duct obstruction
  - Gut perforation (stomach, small intestine, colon)
  - Esophageal perforation
- Medications
  - Drugs causing pancreatitis
  - Sphincter of Oddi spasm
    - Meperidine
    - Codeine
    - Cholinergics
    - Bethanechol
    - Pentazocine
    - Methacholine
    - Morphine
    - Secretin
  - Acetaminophen overdose
  - Valproic acid
- Miscellaneous
  - Renal failure
  - Macrolipasemia
  - Idiopathic
  - Intracranial bleeding
  - Malignancy
  - Hemodialysis

ASCITIC FLUID ANALYSIS

Gross Appearance

- Cloudiness is most often caused by increased neutrophils.
- Bloody specimen may be either due to traumatic tap or nontraumatic causes. Features favoring a traumatic tap include the following:
  - Bloody specimen from a traumatic tap will often clot (nontraumatic bloody ascitic fluid will not clot)
  - Blood associated with a traumatic tap tends to clear with ongoing paracentesis
  - Specimens with blood streaking are more likely due to traumatic taps
- Milky specimen should prompt consideration of chylous or pseudochylous ascites.
- Dark brown specimen should raise concern for biliary or upper gut perforation.
- Black ascites is associated with hemorrhagic pancreatitis and malignant melanoma.

Classification

- Previously, total protein concentration of the ascitic fluid was used to categorize ascites as transudative (<2.5 g/dL) or exudative (>2.5 g/dL).
- In recent years, ascites is best classified using the serum-ascites albumin gradient (SAAG). The SAAG can be calculated by subtracting the ascites albumin concentration from the serum albumin concentration.
- A SAAG >1.1 should prompt consideration of conditions leading to ascites through portal hypertension. These conditions include the following:
  - Cirrhosis
  - Cardiac ascites
  - Alcoholic hepatitis
  - Massive liver metastasis
  - Fulminant hepatic failure
  - Budd-Chiari syndrome
  - Portal vein thrombosis
  - Hepatic veno-occlusive disease
  - Myxedema
  - Acute fatty liver of pregnancy
  - Mixed ascites

- A SAAG <1.1 should prompt consideration of conditions that cause ascites in the absence of portal hypertension. These conditions include the following:
  - Peritoneal carcinomatosis
  - Tuberculous peritonitis
  - Pancreatic ascites
  - Biliary ascites
  - Nephrotic syndrome
  - Serositis (connective tissue disease)
  - Bowel obstruction
  - Bowel infarction
  - Postoperative lymphatic leak

Cell Count

- The reporting of the cell count varies from laboratory to laboratory.
- Some laboratories include mesothelial cells as part of the total white blood cell count, often reporting the sum (mesothelial cells + white blood cells) under the term "nucleated cells".
- Clinical significance of mesothelial cells is unclear.
- White blood cell count is probably the most useful test in the evaluation of ascites because it is the key test needed to exclude infection.
- WBC count in uncomplicated cirrhotic ascites is <500 cells/mm^3.
- Causes of an increased WBC count in the ascitic fluid include the following:
  - Diuresis
  - Spontaneous bacterial peritonitis (SBP)
  - Tuberculous peritonitis
  - Peritoneal carcinomatosis
  - Bloody ascites
  - Chylous ascites
- Predominance of lymphocytes should prompt consideration of tuberculous peritonitis and peritoneal carcinomatosis.

Gram Stain

- Seldom positive
- Positive test result is unusual in SBP and should prompt consideration of very serious infection or gut perforation

Bacterial Culture

- Should be obtained in all patients suspected of having SBP.
- Inoculation of blood culture bottles at the bedside is the preferred method for ascitic fluid culture.

AFB Smear and Culture

- AFB smear is rarely positive.
- Sensitivity of ascitic fluid culture for mycobacteria is about 50%.
- Sensitivity of histology and culture of a peritoneal biopsy is close to 100%.

Cytology

- Overall sensitivity for all types of malignant ascites is 40% to 60%.
- Yield depends upon the mechanism of malignant ascites.
- Sensitivity in patients with peritoneal carcinomatosis is 97%.
- Positive cytology is unlikely if the mechanism of the ascites is extensive liver metastasis or lymphatic obstruction.

Amylase

- An amylase level in normal peritoneal fluid approximates the serum amylase level.
- A rise in the ascitic fluid amylase level (especially if level >3 x normal) is suggestive of pancreatic process (acute pancreatitis, pseudocyst).

Triglyceride Level

- Triglyceride levels should be obtained when milky or opalescent fluid is obtained during paracentesis, raising concern for the possibility of chylous ascites.
- Chylous ascites is the result of lymphatic obstruction and may be due to tumor, trauma, tuberculosis, or filariasis.
- Chylous ascites is typically characterized by triglyceride levels >200 mg/dL.

Bilirubin

- Obtain on ascitic fluid that is brown in color.
- Levels >6 mg/dL should raise concern for biliary or upper gut perforation.

ASCITIC FLUID ANALYSIS

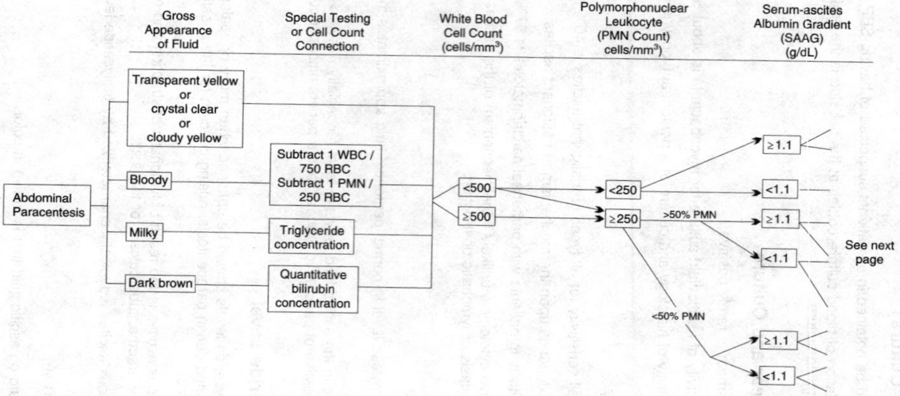
Gross Appearance of Fluid
Special Testing or Cell Count Connection
White Blood Cell Count (cells/mm³)
Polymorphonuclear Leukocyte (PMN Count) cells/mm³)
Serum-ascites Albumin Gradient (SAAG) (g/dL)
Abdominal Paracentesis
Transparent yellow or crystal clear or cloudy yellow
Bloody
Milky
Dark brown
Subtract 1 WBC / 750 RBC Subtract 1 PMN / 250 RBC
Triglyceride concentration
Quantitative bilirubin concentration
<500
≥500
<250
≥250
>50% PMN
<50% PMN
≥1.1
<1.1
≥1.1
<1.1
≥1.1
<1.1
See next page

ASCITIC FLUID ANALYSIS, *continued*

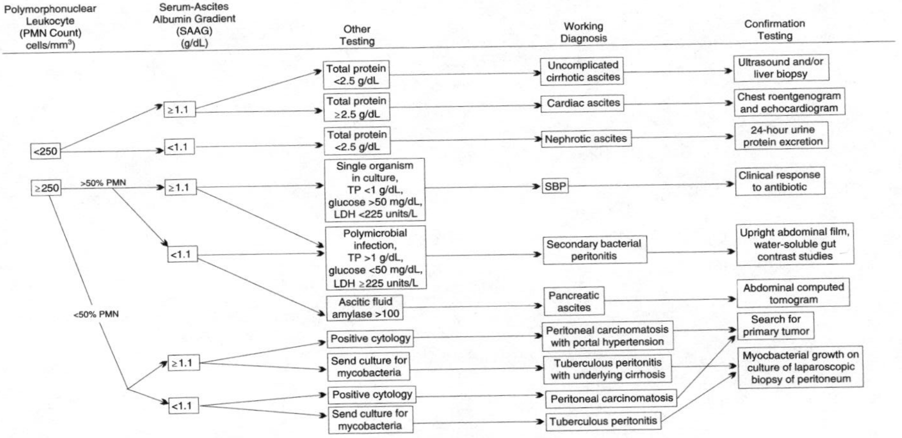
Polymorphonuclear Leukocyte (PMN Count) cells/mm³)
Serum-Ascites Albumin Gradient (SAAG) (g/dL)
Other Testing
Working Diagnosis
Confirmation Testing
<250
≥250
>50% PMN
<50% PMN
≥1.1
<1.1
≥1.1
<1.1
≥1.1
<1.1
Total protein <2.5 g/dL
Total protein ≥2.5 g/dL
Total protein <2.5 g/dL
Single organism in culture, TP <1 g/dL, glucose >50 mg/dL, LDH <225 units/L
Polymicrobial infection, TP >1 g/dL, glucose <50 mg/dL, LDH ≥225 units/L
Ascitic fluid amylase >100
Positive cytology
Send culture for mycobacteria
Positive cytology
Send culture for mycobacteria
Uncomplicated cirrhotic ascites
Cardiac ascites
Nephrotic ascites
SBP
Secondary bacterial peritonitis
Pancreatic ascites
Peritoneal carcinomatosis with portal hypertension
Tuberculous peritonitis with underlying cirrhosis
Peritoneal carcinomatosis
Tuberculous peritonitis
Ultrasound and/or liver biopsy
Chest roentgenogram and echocardiogram
24-hour urine protein excretion
Clinical response to antibiotic
Upright abdominal film, water-soluble gut contrast studies
Abdominal computed tomogram
Search for primary tumor
Myocbacterial growth on culture of laparoscopic biopsy of peritoneum

Adapted from Sleisenger and Fordtrans, *Gastrointesitnal and Liver Disease*, 6th ed, WB Saunders Co, 1998, 1314.

RHEUMATOLOGY

ANTINUCLEAR ANTIBODY

Antinuclear antibodies are antibodies directed against various antigenic material in the nucleus of the cell.

Nuclear Staining Pattern

- The various antinuclear antibodies produce a wide range of nuclear staining patterns depending upon the antigenic material the antibodies are directed against.
- In recent years, the nuclear staining pattern has largely been replaced with assays that determine the type of antibody present.

Type of Antinuclear Antibody

- Antibodies to single- or double-stranded DNA (moderate to high titers): High specificity for SLE
- Antibodies to U1-RNP: Mixed connective tissue disease
- Antibodies to Sm (Smith) antigen: Very specific for SLE (present only in 25% of SLE patients)
- Ro / SSA and La / SSB antibodies: Found with high frequency in Sjögren's syndrome and subacute cutaneous lupus
- Antibodies against Scl-70 (topoisomerase I): Scleroderma
- Anticentromere antibodies: CREST variant of scleroderma
- Antibodies to U3-RNP: Very specific for scleroderma (present only in 10% of scleroderma patients)

Titer of Antibody

- Higher titers of antinuclear antibodies (>1:640) should prompt suspicion for an autoimmune disorder.
- Lower titers may also be significant in patients with signs and symptoms of an autoimmune disorder.
- Lower titers in an asymptomatic patient may be a normal finding.

Causes of Positive ANA

- Connective tissue disease
  - Systemic lupus erythematosus
  - Rheumatoid arthritis
  - Scleroderma
  - Sjögren's syndrome
  - Polymyositis / dermatomyositis
  - Vasculitis
  - Other
- Drug-induced
- Malignancy
  - Lymphoma
  - Leukemia
  - Melanoma
  - Solid cancers (breast, lung)
- Liver disease
  - Chronic active hepatitis
  - Autoimmune hepatitis
  - Primary biliary cirrhosis
- Infection
  - Parasitic
  - Tuberculosis
  - Leprosy
  - *Klebsiella*
  - *Salmonella*
- Pulmonary disease
  - Interstitial pulmonary fibrosis
  - Primary pulmonary hypertension
- Hematologic disorders
  - Idiopathic thrombocytopenic purpura
  - Autoimmune hemolytic anemia
- Endocrine disorders
  - Graves' disease
  - Diabetes mellitus type I

- Multiple sclerosis
- End-stage renal disease
- Status post organ transplantation
- Normal individuals

Evaluation of a Positive ANA

When used in combination with a thorough history and physical examination, interpretation of the ANA may be very useful in confirming or excluding certain diseases. A positive ANA alone does not establish the presence of disease (some healthy individuals have positive ANA, incidence of positive ANA increases with age). By the same token, a negative ANA does not exclude the possibility of autoimmune disease. It must be stressed that ANA results need to be interpreted in relation to the patient's clinical presentation.

Evaluation of a positive ANA in a patient with no apparent rheumatologic or nonrheumatologic condition associated with ANA positivity includes drug history, family history, liver function tests, chest radiograph (to exclude interstitial fibrosis or pulmonary hypertension), CBC (to detect clinically silent hematologic disease), and cultures in the febrile patient. If the cause remains unclear after these studies, then the clinician should follow the patient periodically for the development of one of the above causes of positive ANA.

RHEUMATOID FACTOR

Rheumatoid factor is an antibody directed against the Fc portion of IgG.

Conditions Associated With Positive Rheumatoid Factor

- Aging
- Rheumatologic diseases
  - Rheumatoid arthritis
  - Sjögren's syndrome (75% to 95%)
  - Mixed connective tissue disease (50% to 60%)
  - Mixed cryoglobulinemia types II and III (40% to 100%)
  - Systemic lupus erythematosus (15% to 35%)
  - Polymyositis / dermatomyositis (5% to 10%)
  - Others
- Infection
  - Tuberculosis
  - Subacute bacterial endocarditis
  - Syphilis
  - Leprosy
  - Viral infection
  - Parasitic disease
- Pulmonary
  - Interstitial pulmonary fibrosis
  - Sarcoidosis
  - Asbestosis
  - Silicosis
- Gastrointestinal
  - Primary biliary cirrhosis
  - Chronic viral hepatitis (B or C)
- Miscellaneous
  - Malignancy
  - Following multiple immunizations

SYNOVIAL FLUID ANALYSIS

White Blood Cell Count and Differential

- Normally, synovial fluid has <150 WBC/mm^3 (<25% PMN).
- The total white blood cell count can be used to differentiate inflammatory from noninflammatory arthritis.
- An important cause of inflammatory arthritis that should not be missed is septic arthritis.
  - Many patients with septic arthritis have total WBC counts >100,000/mm^3 and the differential count classically reveals >95% neutrophils.
  - Some (immunocompromised patients, gonococcal infection, partially treated bacterial arthritis), however, have lower degrees of elevation and sometimes, it can be difficult to differentiate septic arthritis from other causes of inflammatory arthritis (ie, gout) in these patients.
  - In addition to the white blood cell count and differential, it is important to obtain Gram stain and culture (perform blood cultures as well as cultures at any other appropriate site).

Crystals

- In patients with acute gouty arthritis, crystals are seen in approximately 90% of cases. Monosodium urate crystals are characteristically negatively birefringent and needle-shaped.
- The crystals (calcium pyrophosphate dihydrate) of pseudogout are rhomboid-shaped and demonstrate weakly positive birefringence
- It is important to realize that both septic arthritis and crystal-induced arthritis can occur together.

Gram Stain / Culture

- If there is any suspicion for bacterial arthritis (septic arthritis), Gram stain and culture should be obtained.
- The yield is higher if these studies are obtained before starting antibiotic therapy.
- The likelihood of having positive test results depends on a variety of factors, including the etiologic organism (yield is usually lower with gonococcal arthritis).
- Studies for tuberculosis and fungal organisms should not be routinely done but if there is suspicion for this type of infection, then appropriate studies should be performed (acid-fast smear, cultures, etc).

CARDIOLOGY

CARDIAC ENZYMES

Cardiac enzymes are most often obtained in the evaluation of the patient suspected of having an acute myocardial infarction. Cardiac enzymes include the following:

- Creatine kinase
- Troponin
- Myoglobin

World Health Organization Criteria for the Diagnosis of Acute Myocardial Infarction

- Many years ago, the WHO established three criteria for the diagnosis of acute myocardial infarction:
  - Chest pain or discomfort consistent with acute myocardial infarction
  - EKG findings consistent with acute myocardial infarction
  - Characteristic elevation of the cardiac enzymes
- The diagnosis of acute myocardial infarction required two of the three criteria to be fulfilled
- In recent years, we have realized that many patients with acute myocardial infarction present with nonspecific EKG changes; some even have no EKG abnormalities suggestive of acute myocardial infarction
- Other patients may not present with the typical symptoms of acute myocardial infarction; some even have silent myocardial infarction
- Because of the limitations of the clinical presentation and EKG findings in the diagnosis of acute myocardial infarction, clinicians are relying more heavily on cardiac enzyme testing

Troponin

- Troponin is now the cardiac enzyme of choice in the evaluation of patients suspected of having myocardial infarction
- Troponin is very specific for myocardial injury
- Troponin typically rises 4-6 hours after onset but may remain elevated for up to 10 days
- Because troponin levels may remain elevated for prolonged period of time, it can be difficult to determine when the ischemic event took place if the clinician relies on the troponin level alone. For this reason, CK-MB levels should be

obtained. CK-MB remains elevated for up to 48 hours. Therefore, when both CK-MB and troponin levels are elevated, the clinician can be more confident of a recent acute myocardial infarction.

- Normal CK-MB levels in the patient with an elevated troponin level should prompt consideration of an event that was not so recent (>48 hours prior to presentation)
- In patients with unstable angina, troponin elevation has been shown to be an independent risk factor for future ischemic events

Creatine Kinase

- Creatine kinase elevation lacks specificity for cardiac injury because it is present elsewhere in the body (in addition to cardiac muscle)
- Specificity of the creatine kinase can be improved by measuring the MB fraction (see below)
- Most patients have an increased creatine kinase four to six hours after the onset of the acute myocardial infarction
- Some, however, may not have an increase until twelve hours after onset
- Peak levels are reached 18-24 hours after onset
- Creatine kinase levels return to normal 48 hours after onset
- False-positive test results can occur with skeletal muscle injury or central nervous system disease

MB Fraction of Creatine Kinase (CK-MB)

- CK-MB is more specific for cardiac injury when compared to creatine kinase
- Similar to the creatine kinase, CK-MB rises 4-6 hours after onset of acute myocardial infarction
- Some, however, may not have an increase in the CK-MB until twelve hours after onset
- Rise and fall of the CK-MB in the patient who has a clinical presentation compatible with myocardial infarction is the key to establishing the diagnosis
- CK-MB levels may also rise due to skeletal muscle injury
- When CK-MB rises due to skeletal muscle injury, the rise in the CK-MB tends to be slower and the plateau of CK-MB elevation is more sustained. In addition, the fall in the CK-MB levels is slower as well.

Myoglobin

- Myoglobin is an oxygen binding protein that is released from myocardial cells when they are injured
- Because it has the lowest molecular weight of all the cardiac enzymes, it is released into the circulation first.
- It can be detected 1-4 hours after the insult
- Myoglobin level peaks at 4-12 hours
- It is cleared from the circulation within 24 hours

COST-EFFECTIVE WORK-UP FOR ACUTE CHEST PAIN

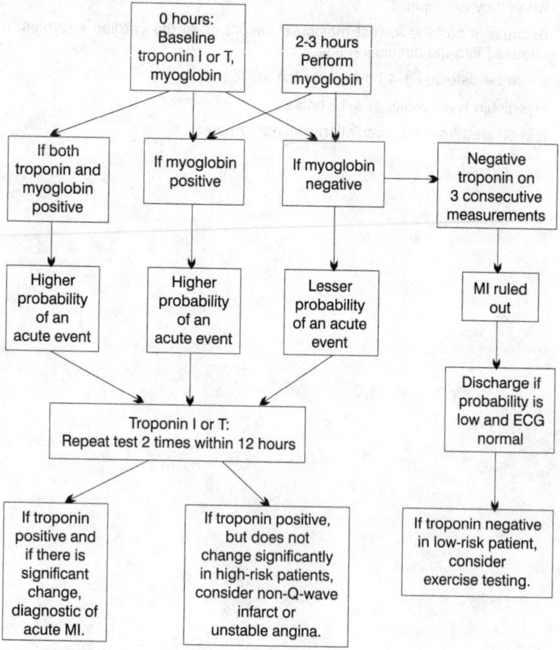
0 hours:
Baseline
troponin I or T,
myoglobin
2-3 hours
Perform
myoglobin
If both
troponin and
myoglobin
positive
If myoglobin
positive
If myoglobin
negative
Negative
troponin on
3 consecutive
measurements
Higher
probability
of an
acute event
Higher
probability
of an
acute event
Lesser
probability
of an acute
event
MI ruled
out
Discharge if
probability is
low and ECG
normal
Troponin I or T:
Repeat test 2 times within 12 hours
If troponin
positive and
if there is
significant
change,
diagnostic of
acute MI.
If troponin positive,
but does not
change significantly
in high-risk patients,
consider non-Q-wave
infarct or
unstable angina.
If troponin negative
in low-risk patient,
consider
exercise testing.

ECG = electrocardiogram
MI = myocardial infarction

Adapted from Khan F, Sachs HJ, Pechet L, et al, *Guide to Diagnostic Testing*, Philadelphia, PA: Lippincott Williams & Wilkins, 2002, 35.

LIPID PROFILE

Fasting Versus Nonfasting Measurement

- Standard lipid profile consists of the following:
  - Total cholesterol
  - HDL-cholesterol
  - Triglyceride
- LDL-cholesterol is not usually measured but calculated according to the following formula:
  - LDL-cholesterol = Total cholesterol - VLDL - HDL where VLDL = triglyceride / 5
  - One limitation of this formula is that it loses its validity if triglyceride levels exceed 400 mg/dL
  - When triglyceride level >400 mg/dL, it is better to measure LDL directly
- Effects of fasting on the components of the lipid profile
  - Serum total cholesterol and HDL-cholesterol can be measured fasting or nonfasting; very little difference between the two
  - Triglyceride level is affected by recent eating

Measuring Lipid Levels in the Hospital

- Lipid levels may be affected by the acute phase response that is associated with certain conditions such as myocardial infarction, surgery, trauma, or infection
  - Total cholesterol, HDL-cholesterol, and LDL-cholesterol may decline
  - Triglyceride level usually rises
- Hospitalization, even in the absence of the acute phase response, has been shown to lower HDL-cholesterol levels
- For these reasons, it is preferable to delay lipoprotein analysis for one to two months after discharge

National Cholesterol Education Program Guidelines

- NCEP III recommend cholesterol screening once every 5 years in those over the age of 20
- Guidelines recommend fasting lipid profile for screening
- If nonfasting lipid profile is obtained, total cholesterol >200 mg/dL or HDL <40 mg/dL should prompt performance of fasting lipid profile

- If no coronary heart disease (CHD), desirable serum LDL concentration for patient with no or one risk factor for CHD is <160 mg/dL - if desirable serum LDL concentration met, then repeat screening is recommended in 5 years
- If no CHD, desirable serum LDL concentration for patient with two or more risk factors for CHD is <130 mg/dL - if desirable serum LDL concentration met, then repeat screening is recommended in 5 years
- Desirable serum LDL-cholesterol concentration is <100 mg/dL in the following groups of patients:
  - CHD
  - Diabetes mellitus
  - Abdominal aortic aneurysm
  - Peripheral arterial disease
  - Symptomatic carotid artery disease

Approach to the Patient With Hypertriglyceridemia

- Triglyceride levels <150 mg/dL are considered normal
- Triglyceride levels between 150-200 mg/dL are considered borderline high
- Triglyceride levels 200-499 mg/dL are considered high
- Triglyceride levels >500 mg/dL are considered very high
- Every patient with hypertriglyceridemia should be evaluated for conditions that predispose to higher triglyceride levels. Conditions that should be considered include:
  - Obesity
  - Diabetes mellitus (obtain plasma glucose)
  - Nephrotic syndrome (obtain urinalysis)
  - Renal failure (obtain serum creatinine)
  - Estrogen replacement
  - Hypothyroidism (obtain thyroid function tests)
  - Medications (β-blockers, glucocorticoids, cyclosporine, thiazides, loop diuretics, ticlid)

TOPIC INDEX

A

G

H

NOTES

NOTES

NOTES

NOTES

NOTES

NOTES

Other titles offered by Lexi-Comp, Inc.

DRUG INTERACTIONS HANDBOOK

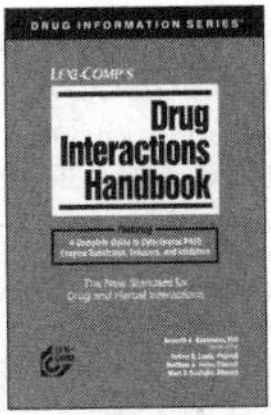
DRUG INFORMATION SERIES
LEXI-COMP'S
Drug Interactions Handbook

Perfect Bound / Book Size: 5.5" x 8.5"

by Bachmann, Lewis, Fuller, Bonfiglio

The New Standard for Evaluating Drug and Herbal Interactions

A comprehensive table of Cytochrome P450 enzyme substrates, inducers and inhibitors. Each interaction monograph contains the following ratings: **Reliability Rating** - indicating the quantity and nature of documentation for an interaction: **A** - No Known Interaction, **B** - No Action Needed, **C** - Monitor Therapy, **D** - Consider Therapy Modification, and **X** - Avoid Combination; **Severity Rating** - indicating the reported or possible magnitude of an interaction outcome.

DRUG INFORMATION HANDBOOK FOR THE ALLIED HEALTH PROFESSIONAL

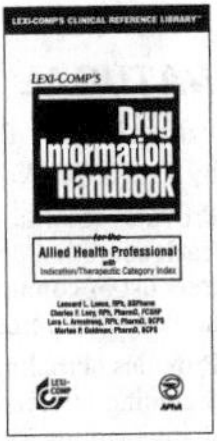
LEXI-COMP'S CLINICAL REFERENCE LIBRARY
LEXI-COMP'S
Drug Information Handbook
Allied Health Professional

Perfect Bound / Book Size: 4.5" x 9"

by Lance, Lacy, Armstrong, Goldman

Working with clinical pharmacists, hospital pharmacy and therapeutics committees, and hospital drug information centers, the authors have assisted hundreds of hospitals in developing institution-specific formulary reference documentation. The most current basic drug and medication data from those clinical settings have been reviewed, coalesced, and cross-referenced to create this unique handbook. The handbook offers quick access to abbreviated monographs for generic drugs. This is a great tool for physician assistants, medical records personnel, medical transcriptionists and secretaries, pharmacy technicians, and other allied health professionals.

PHARMACOGENOMICS HANDBOOK

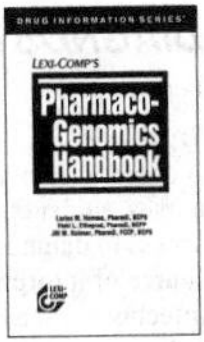
DRUG INFORMATION SERIES
LEXI-COMP'S
Pharmaco-Genomics Handbook

Perfect Bound / Book Size: 4.25" x 7"

by Humma, Ellingrod, Kolesar

This exciting new title by Lexi-Comp, introduces Pharmacogenomics to the forward-thinking healthcare professional and student! It presents information concerning key genetic variations that may influence drug disposition and/or sensitivity. Brief introductions to fundamental concepts in genetics and genomics are provided in order to bring the reader up-to-date on these rapidly emerging sciences. This book provides a foundation for all clinicians who will be called on to integrate rapidly expanding genomic knowledge into the management of drug therapy. A great introduction to pharmacogenetic principles as well as a concise reference on key polymorphisms known to influence drug response!

To order call toll free anywhere in the U.S.: 1-800-837-LEXI (5394)

Outside of the U.S. call: 330-650-6506 or online at www.lexi.com

Other titles offered by Lexi-Comp, Inc.

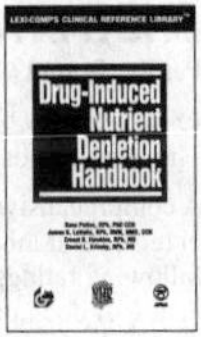
Drug-Induced
Nutrient
Depletion
Handbook

DRUG-INDUCED NUTRIENT DEPLETION HANDBOOK

Perfect Bound / Book Size: 4.25" x 7"

by Pelton, LaValle, Hawkins, Krinsky

A complete and up-to-date listing of all drugs known to deplete the body of nutritional compounds. This book is alphabetically organized and provides extensive cross-referencing to related information in the various sections of the book. Drug monographs identify the nutrients depleted and provide cross-references to the nutrient monographs for more detailed information on effects of depletion, biological function & effect, side effects & toxicity, RDA, dosage range, and dietary sources. this book also contains a studies & abstracts section, a valuable appendix, and alphabetical & pharmacological indexes.

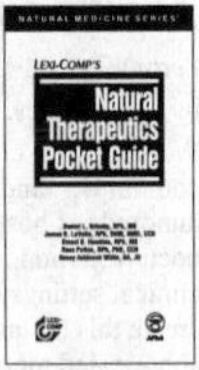
LEXI-COMP'S
Natural
Therapeutics
Pocket Guide

NATURAL THERAPEUTICS POCKET GUIDE

Perfect Bound / Book Size: 4.375" x 8"

by Krinsky, LaValle, Hawkins, Pelton, Ashbrook Willis

Provides condition-specific information on common uses of natural therapies. Each condition discussed includes the following: review of condition, decision tree, list of commonly recommended herbals, nutritional supplements, homeopathic remedies, lifestyle modifications, and special considerations. Provides herbal/nutritional/nutraceutical monographs with over 10 fields including references, reported uses, dosage, pharmacology, toxicity, warnings & interactions, and cautions & contraindications. The Appendix includes: drug-nutrient depletion, herb-drug interactions, drug-nutrient interaction, herbal medicine use in pediatrics, unsafe herbs, and reference of top herbals.

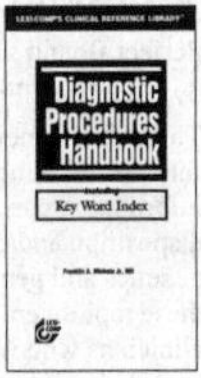
Diagnostic
Procedures
Handbook
Key Word Index

DIAGNOSTIC PROCEDURES HANDBOOK

Perfect Bound / Book Size: 4.375" x 8"

by Michota

A comprehensive, yet concise, quick reference source for physicians, nurses, students, medical records personnel, or anyone needing quick access to diagnostic procedure information. This handbook is an excellent source of information in the following areas: allergy, rheumatology, and infectious disease; cardiology; computed tomography; diagnostic radiology; gastroenterology; invasive radiology; magnetic resonance imaging; nephrology, urology, and hematology; neurology; nuclear medicine; pulmonary function; pulmonary medicine and critical care; ultrasound; and women's health.

To order call toll free anywhere in the U.S.: 1-800-837-LEXI (5394)

Outside of the U.S. call: 330-650-6506 or online at www.lexi.com

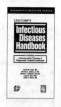

Other titles offered by Lexi-Comp, Inc.

CLINICIAN'S GUIDE TO INTERNAL MEDICINE—A Practical Approach

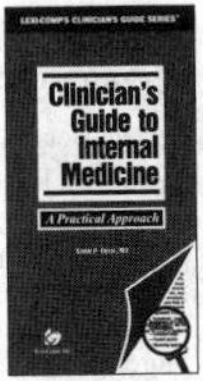
Clinician's Guide to Internal Medicine
A Practical Approach

Perfect Bound / Book Size: 4.375" x 8"

by Desai

Provides quick access to essential information covering diagnosis, treatment, and management of commonly encountered patient problems in Internal Medicine. This up-to-date and clinically-relevant information is in an easy-to-read format and is easily accessible. Provides practical approaches that are not readily available in standard textbooks. Contains algorithms to help you establish the diagnosis and select the appropriate therapy. There are numerous tables and boxes that summarize diagnostic and therapeutic strategies. An ideal reference for use at the point-of-care. This is a reference companion that will provide you with the tools necessary to tackle even the most challenging problems in Internal Medicine.

CLINICIAN'S GUIDE TO DIAGNOSIS —A Practical Approach

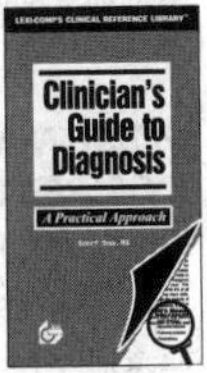
Clinician's Guide to Diagnosis
A Practical Approach

Perfect Bound / Book Size: 4.375" x 8"

by Desai

Symptoms are what prompt patients to seek medical care. In the evaluation of a patient's symptom, it is not unusual for healthcare professionals to ask "What do I do next?" This is precisely the question for which this book provides the answer. It will lead you from symptom to diagnosis through a series of steps designed to mimic the logical thought processes of seasoned clinicians. For the young clinician, this is an ideal book to help bridge the gap between the classroom and actual patient care. For the experienced clinician, this concise handbook offers rapid answers to the questions that are commonly encountered on a day-to-day basis. Let this guide become your companion, providing you with the tools necessary to tackle even the most challenging symptoms.

CLINICIAN'S GUIDE TO LABORATORY MEDICINE—A Practical Approach

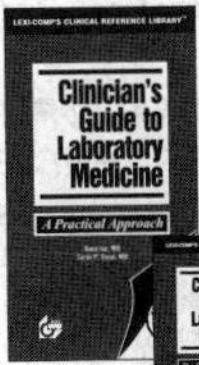
Clinician's Guide to Laboratory Medicine
A Practical Approach

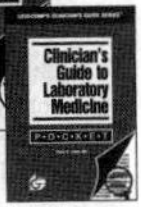
Clinician's Guide to Laboratory Medicine
POCKET

Perfect Bound / Book Size: 4.375" x 8" Pocket Guide: 4.25" x 7"

by Desai, Isa-Pratt

When faced with abnormal laboratory tests, the clinician can now turn to the this source for it's unique ability to lead the clinician from laboratory test abnormality to clinical diagnosis. Written for the busy clinician, this concise handbook will provide rapid answers to the questions that busy clinicians face in the care of their patients. No longer does the clinician have to struggle in an effort to find this information - it's all here. A **FREE copy** of the *Pocket* sized guide included.

To order call toll free anywhere in the U.S.: 1-800-837-LEXI (5394)

Outside of the U.S. call: 330-650-6506 or online at www.lexi.com

Other titles offered by Lexi-Comp, Inc.

LABORATORY TEST HANDBOOK & CONCISE Edition

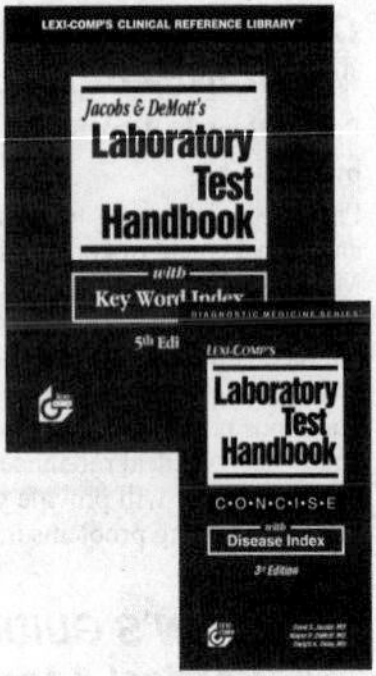
LEXI-COMP'S CLINICAL REFERENCE LIBRARY
Jacobs & DeMott's
Laboratory Test Handbook
with
DIAGNOSTIC MEDICINE SERIES
LEXI-COMP'S
Laboratory Test Handbook
C·O·N·C·I·S·E
with
Disease Index

Perfect Bound / Book Size: 8.5" x 11" Concise: 4.375" x 8"

by Jacobs, DeMott, Oxley

Contains over 900 clinical laboratory tests and is an excellent source of laboratory information for physicians of all specialties, nurses, laboratory professionals, students, medical personnel, or anyone who needs quick access to most routine and many of the more specialized testing procedures available in today's clinical laboratory. Each monograph contains test name, synonyms, patient care, specimen requirements, reference ranges, and interpretive information with footnotes, references, and selected web sites.

The *Laboratory Test Handbook Concise* is a portable, abridged (800 tests) version and is an ideal, quick reference for anyone requiring information concerning patient preparation, specimen collection and handling, and test result interpretation.

POISONING & TOXICOLOGY COMPENDIUM

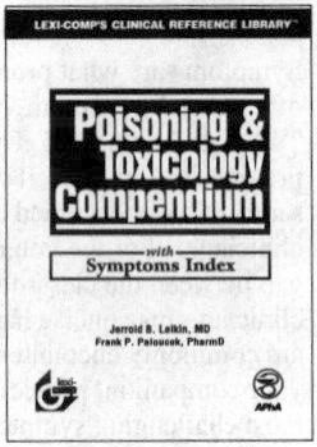
LEXI-COMP'S CLINICAL REFERENCE LIBRARY
Poisoning & Toxicology Compendium
with
Symptoms Index
Jerrold B. Leikin, MD
Frank P. Paloucek, PharmD
APhA

Case Bound / Book Size: 8.5" x 11"

by Leikin and Paloucek

A six-in-one reference wherein each major entry contains information relative to one or more of the other sections. This compendium offers comprehensive, concisely-stated monographs covering 645 medicinal agents, 256 nonmedicinal agents, 273 biological agents, 49 herbal agents, 254 laboratory tests, 79 antidotes, and 222 pages of exceptionally useful appendix material.

A truly unique reference that presents signs and symptoms of acute overdose along with considerations for overdose treatment. Ideal reference for emergency situations.

DENTAL OFFICE MEDICAL EMERGENCIES

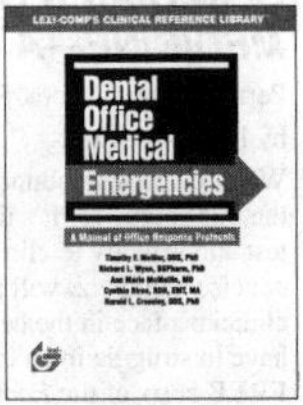
LEXI-COMP'S CLINICAL REFERENCE LIBRARY
Dental Office Medical Emergencies
A Manual of Office Response Protocols

Spiral Bound / Book Size: 8.5" x 11"

by Meiller, Wynn, McMullin, Crossley

Designed specifically for general dentists during times of emergency. A tabbed paging system allows for quick access to specific crisis events. Created with urgency in mind, it is spiral bound and drilled with a hole for hanging purposes.

To order call toll free anywhere in the U.S.: 1-800-837-LEXI (5394)

Outside of the U.S. call: 330-650-6506 or online at www.lexi.com

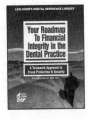

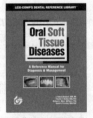

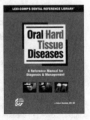

Other titles offered by Lexi-Comp, Inc.

PATIENT EDUCATION
Wall Posters

Ideal for Waiting Rooms and Examination Rooms.

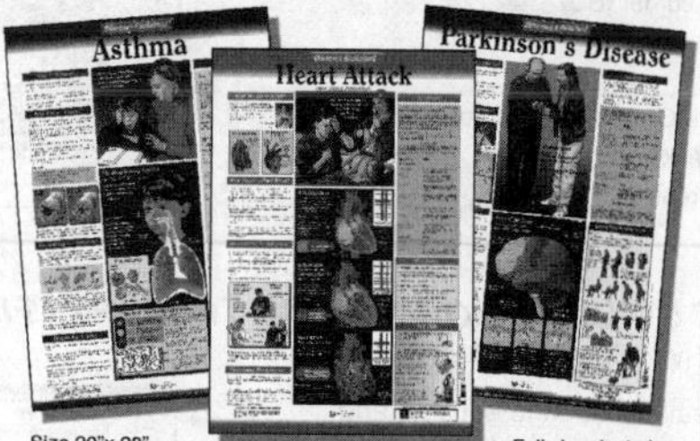
Asthma
Heart Attack
Parkinson's Disease

Size 20"x 28" — Fully Laminated

Written in a layman's language and presented in an easy-to-follow, graphic style. Each condition is carefully described, along with the treatments available, and complex medical terms are explained.

Titles available

Acne	*Heart Attack*
Alzheimer's Disease	*HIV and AIDS*
Anemia	*Hypertension*
Angina	*Irritable Bowel Syndrome*
Anxiety	*Incontinence*
Asthma	*Insomnia*
Bipolar Disorder	*Menopause*
Breast Cancer	*Migraine*
Congestive Heart Failure	*Multiple Sclerosis*
Cholesterol	*OCD*
COPD	*Osteoporosis*
Depression	*Otitis Media*
Diabetes	*Panic Attacks*
Deep Vein Thrombosis	*Parkinson's Disease*
Enlarged Prostate (BPH)	*Schizophrenia*
Epilepsy	*Spasticity*
Essential Tremor	*Stroke*
Glaucoma	*Thyroid Disease*

To order a catalog, call Toll Free at: 1-877-837-5394
or visit us online at - **www.diseases-explained.com**

Diseases Explained ™

DXLX04/1

To order call toll free anywhere in the U.S.: 1-800-837-LEXI (5394)
Outside of the U.S. call: 330-650-6506 or online at www.lexi.com